Health is the most precious thing you can possess. And when your health is good, you feel vibrant and alive. You deserve to have all the energy you need for work, play, family—everything in your life. Our goal is to get you there, by first showing you what may be holding you back, then outlining a healthy way to live, and finally putting it all together in an easy-to-do Three-Week Plan. It has worked for us and our patients, and it will work for you. Enjoy the journey!

Dr. Peter Bennett

Dr. Stephen Barrie

Contents

This book is organized into three sections: the first describes the problem, the second outlines the solution and the third puts it all together in the Three-Week Plan. Feel free to jump around! Read the parts that apply to you the most. When you're ready to start the Plan, go for it. You can always go back to the first two sections for inspiration and guidance.

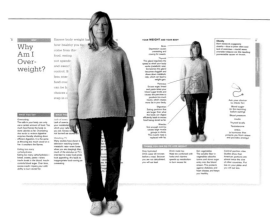

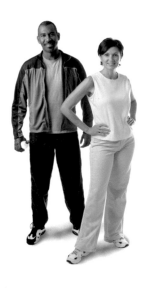

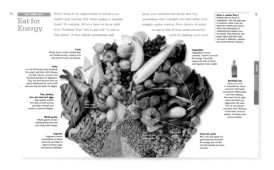

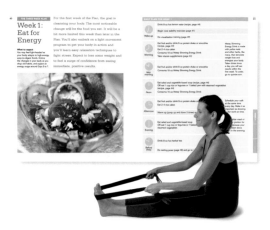

FATIGUED

OVERWEIGHT

STRESSED

EATING

MOVING

RELAXING

WEEK 1

WEEK 2

WEEK 3

If you want to improve your health, you really are asking to take control of three things: your energy, your weight and your stress level. And you can. But first you need to clearly see what has thrown one, two or all three of these elements out of balance.

Change Begins with Asking Why

To get started, let's look at where you are right now. What choices are you making that contribute to feeling stressed, fatigued or overweight? How are these three factors affecting your overall health? Once you understand what is going on, we will show you what you can do: make choices that boost your health and your energy. It's not as hard as you might think. This section will show you what to change and, in the rest of the book, we'll tell you how.

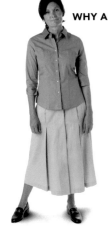

WHY AM I **TIRED?**

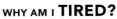

WHY AM I **OVERWEIGHT?**

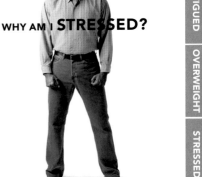

WHY AM I **STRESSED?**

Do you wake up tired or feeling like you need more sleep? Do you run out of energy every afternoon? Do you need to nap when you come home from work? In this section, you will learn what factors make you feel tired, how this fatigue affects your overall health and what you can do about it to boost your energy.

Have you been struggling to lose those extra 10 pounds for the past six months? Are you constantly jumping on and off different diets with little or no success? Take a look at how the things you eat, do and feel influence your body. You'll see how making good choices can give you back control of your weight.

Do you feel panicky, unfocused or overwhelmed? Do you get depressed, frustrated or lose your temper easily? Stress has a huge impact on every aspect of your health. In this section you'll come to understand the stressors in your life and how to manage them to feel less stressed.

Why Am I Tired?

You aren't "just tired." It's more than that. Feeling a lack of energy is the most basic way your body tells you that something is out of balance. Your energy level is related to every system in your body and to everything you eat and do. Even small and simple changes can give you an immediate boost. Look at all the factors that drain your vitality so you can make energy-enhancing choices.

WHAT YOU EAT

Nutrient deficient diet
Foods that are high in sugar and refined flour, most snacks, sweets and fast food, fill you up without giving your body what it needs for energy. These foods throw off the body's ability to regulate blood sugar. The resulting low blood sugar is called hypoglycemia and causes sluggishness and irritability.

Food allergies
For many people, certain foods like wheat and dairy products can cause allergic symptoms like fatigue, headaches, joint pain and frequent colds. The body's energy is drained by constantly going through an allergic reaction.

Dehydration
Not drinking enough water thickens the blood, which is mostly water. Thicker blood circulates more slowly and carries nutrients to your cells less effectively.

WHAT YOU DO

Lack of exercise and toxicity
The act of moving your body and using your muscles helps eliminate toxins—chemicals in our body that can't be used and can interfere with cell function. Exercise helps to circulate and remove waste products from your cells. In a body that doesn't move enough, the toxins linger and accumulate.

Lack of exercise and mood
Exercise stimulates the production of endorphins in the brain. These are "feel-good chemicals" which give a natural sense of well-being and energy. Without them, you feel tired and depressed.

Lack of exercise and metabolism
Lack of exercise lowers your metabolic rate, the speed at which your body operates and produces energy. The lower the rate, the less efficiently your body will convert the food you eat into energy for your cells, organs and brain.

WHAT YOU FEEL

Stress
Stress makes you feel tired and overwhelmed because it releases the stress hormone cortisol. This chemical puts the body in a state of emergency which, when sustained over time, causes exhaustion.

Poor sleep
Without sufficient sleep, the nervous system cannot regenerate itself, replenish lost energy reserves in brain cells and restore chemical balance.

Negative emotions
Negative emotions cause the brain to produce adrenaline, the emergency "fight or flight" hormone. This depletes available blood sugar and leads to a "sugar crash," a sudden lack of energy.

FATIGUE AND YOUR BODY

Blood
Poor blood oxygenation from not enough exercise reduces energy.

Lungs
Lack of exercise reduces oxygen intake and makes you feel worn out.

Heart
Being overweight makes the heart work less efficiently, making you tired.

Liver
Toxins from food and the environment overwhelm the liver's ability to purify the blood.

Adrenal glands
Too much stress weakens the adrenal glands.

Digestion
Food allergies and imbalance in stomach acid (caused by stress or genetic factors) prevent efficient conversion of food into energy.

Immune system
Food allergies cause overload, making your system work harder.

Hormones
Stress hormones lower the levels of energy hormones like thyroid, DHEA and testosterone.

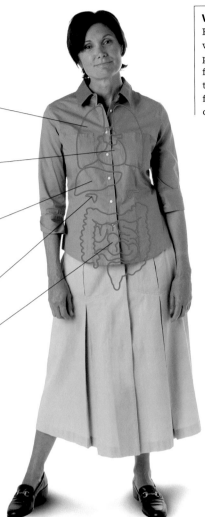

What is "chronic fatigue"?
Extreme tiredness, along with other symptoms like pain, loss of mental focus and frequent illness, could be the condition called chronic fatigue syndrome. It is a result of multiple system failure.

Ask your doctor to check for:

Anemia (not enough healthy red blood cells)

Thyroid levels

Low cortisol

Food allergies

Heavy metal toxicity (mercury, lead)

Chronic viral infection

THINGS YOU CAN DO TO IMPROVE YOUR ENERGY LEVEL

Eliminate food allergens
Get tested for allergies or avoid common allergy-causing foods (such as dairy) for a while to see if it changes your energy level.

Supplement your food intake
Nutritional supplements and energy drinks stimulate cellular function to increase energy production.

Regulate stress hormones
You can control your hormone levels by controlling your stress levels. Taking time to relax each day reduces the exhaustion that comes from stress.

Get more sleep
Give yourself at least 8 hours of restful sleep each night to rejuvenate your mind and body. Short-changing yourself on sleep leads to exhaustion.

Why Am I Over-weight?

Excess body weight has a huge impact on how healthy you feel. Those extra pounds come from three factors: eating too much food, eating food from the wrong sources and not spending enough energy in movement and exercise. All three factors are under your control. But extra weight can make you feel less energetic and more inclined to choose food over exercise. It is a cycle, but one that can be broken. Take a look at how your daily choices affect your weight—that's the first step in regaining control of it.

WHAT YOU EAT

Overeating
The cells in your body can only use a certain amount of food. Too much food forces the body to store calories as fat. Overeating also tends to reduce digestive enzymes thereby shutting down efficient digestion. It is the same as throwing too much wood on a fire: it smothers the flames.

Eating too many carbohydrates
Eating too many carbohydrates—bread, sweets, pasta—raises insulin levels in the blood. Insulin controls blood sugar. Over time, excess insulin impairs your cells' ability to burn stored fat.

WHAT YOU DO

Lack of exercise
Lack of exercise slows down your metabolism—the rate at which your cells use the food you eat. Excess calories that are not burned are stored as fat.

Watching TV
Many studies have shown that television watching lowers metabolic rate—even lower than when you are sleeping! Also, much of the stimulus on TV is intended to make food products look appealing; this leads to inappropriate food craving and overeating.

WHAT YOU FEEL

Depression
Depression can cause inactivity, night eating and overeating.

Winter darkness
For some people, lack of sunlight during winter months causes Seasonal Affective Disorder (SAD), an imbalance of the brain hormones that regulate mood. SAD can resemble depression and so it, too, can cause weight gain.

Negative emotions
Negative emotions like poor self-esteem cause stress. To deal with the stress, the body produces stress hormones that eventually lower blood sugar levels and cause inactivity, which leads to weight gain.

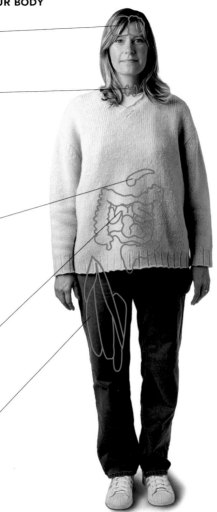

Brain
Depression causes overeating and craving for sweets.

Thyroid
This gland regulates the speed at which your body works (metabolic rate). Sometimes this gland becomes sluggish and slows down metabolic rate, which can lead to weight gain.

Pancreas
Excess sugar, bread and pasta raises your blood sugar levels and causes the pancreas to produce too much insulin, which creates more fat in your body.

Digestion
Eating portions that are larger than what the body can digest efficiently leads to excess food being stored as fat.

Muscles
Not enough exercise causes large muscle groups to shrink. This muscle mass is replaced with fat.

Obesity
New research suggests obesity—due to poor diet and lack of exercise—could soon overtake tobacco as the leading preventable cause of death.

Ask your doctor to check for:

Blood sugar (in the morning before eating)

Blood pressure

Insulin

Thyroid levels

Testosterone

DHEA (a hormone that protects you from stress and provides energy)

THINGS YOU CAN DO TO LOSE WEIGHT

Stay hydrated
Drink water 20 minutes before a meal. Because you are not dehydrated, you will eat less!

.

Drink maté tea
Maté tea combined with herbs and vitamins speeds up metabolism to burn excess fat.

Eat vegetables
The soluble fiber in vegetables absorbs toxins and slows sugar entry into the blood stream. This protects against diabetes and heart disease, and keeps you healthy.

Control portion size
Studies show that American portions are almost twice the size of other countries. Put less on your plate and you will eat less.

Why Am I Stressed?

Stress can come from many different sources. Whether you have financial difficulties, a boss who doesn't treat you well, an injury or a difficult relationship, your body tries to deal with it all in the same way: by producing stress hormones. These chemicals rev up your body at first, but eventually deplete your energy. When you get exhausted in this way, it becomes even harder to deal with the stressors in your life. Because stress is very individual, learn to recognize the things that cause you stress, and make choices that minimize their impact on your health.

WHAT YOU EAT

Too much sugar
Stress hormones raise your blood sugar levels. This can lead to sugar craving. Eating sugar repeats the cycle by sending more stress signals to the body.

Not enough healthy fats
The "good" fat found in fish and fish oil is vital for health. It strengthens the membranes of your cells and helps to keep in balance high blood sugar caused by stress.

Food allergies
Eating foods you are allergic to stimulates the production of adrenaline, a hormone that revs up your body. This causes anxiety and, over time, exhaustion.

WHAT YOU DO

Too little or no exercise
Proper exercise relaxes the nervous system, lowers blood pressure, regulates the heart rate and opens up circulation. All these send a message to the brain that it can relax.

Excessive exercise
Too much exercise causes wear and tear and injuries. Too vigorous exercise causes the body to produce stress hormones.

Keeping up
Trying to match the fast pace of everyday life—traffic, deadlines, workloads, family duties—increases stress levels.

WHAT YOU FEEL

Financial difficulties
A mortgage or rent you can't afford causes your body to make the same stress hormones you would produce if you were in a fight or flight situation such as being chased by a bear.

Personal problems with friends and family
The nervous system responds to stressful relationships and produces chemicals that alter blood sugar and insulin levels.

Feeling stuck, alone or depressed
Having the perception of being trapped is an important signal to the brain. The more "inescapable" your situation seems, the more stress hormones you will produce.

STRESS AND YOUR BODY

Brain
Stress disturbs the healthy balance of neurotransmitters in the brain.

Thyroid
Under chronic stress, the thyroid gland shuts down and fails to regulate how your body uses fuel.

Heart
Heart rate is elevated by stress, causing it to work harder and less efficiently.

Adrenal glands
Small adrenal glands on top of the kidneys produce over 50 hormones. When triggered repeatedly by stress they disturb the balance of other hormones, including thyroid, insulin, testosterone and estrogen.

Muscles and joints
Chronic pain in muscles and joints can be both a cause and a symptom of stress.

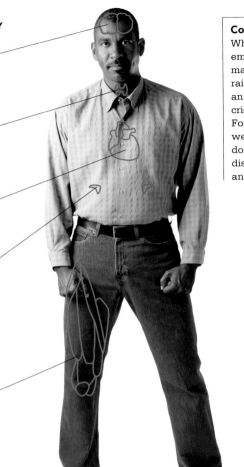

Cortisol: the stress hormone
When you are faced with an emergency, your adrenal gland makes cortisol. This hormone raises blood sugar to give you an energy boost. In a short-term crisis, this could help you survive. For the long-term situations we have in modern life, cortisol does more harm than good: it disturbs sleep, disrupts memory and impairs immune functions.

Ask your doctor to check for:

Anemia

Blood pressure

Blood sugar
(in the morning before eating)

Food allergies

Heavy metal toxicity
(mercury, lead)

Cortisol

Thyroid levels

STRESSED

THINGS YOU CAN DO TO DECREASE STRESS

Relax
Use breathing techniques, visualization, movement, positive thinking and yoga to help you relax.

Slow down
Take charge of your life's pace by making time for relaxation. It balances emotions and reduces stress.

.

Heal chronic pain
Get massage, chiropractic or physical therapy for nagging aches and pains.

Make a life plan
Write down goals for your job, relationships, money and future. This will help you remain realistic and meet your expectations.

Now that you have taken a look at how you feel and why, you are ready to take the next step. In this section, you will learn a few simple principles about what to eat, how to move your body and how to relax. You can unlock your energized life

Three Keys to Healthy Living

only if you make changes to all three essential keys to health: eating, moving and relaxing. The best part, as our patients quickly learn, is that each key encourages the others: moving your body makes you want to eat right; energizing food makes you want to take the time to relax; stress reduction encourages restful sleep so you feel ready to exercise. All three keys work together to improve your energy, weight and stress level.

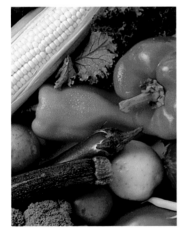

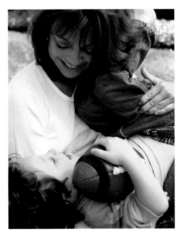

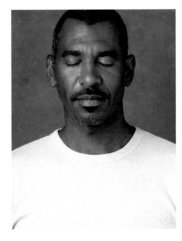

Food and eating

What you eat, how much you eat and how you prepare your food all have a huge impact on your health. In this section, you will see which foods energize you and which ones slow you down. You'll learn ways to prepare great-tasting meals that boost energy and help you control your weight.

Moving and activity

Your body is made to move. Even the simplest movement— taking a walk—stimulates every part of your body to work better. There is no pill, vitamin or food that can take the place of walking, stretching and breathing. Find out how putting your body into daily action benefits you.

Relaxation and stress reduction

It may seem like it's all in your mind, but stress affects your body just as dramatically as pain or injury. Relaxing for even a short time each day recharges and energizes your entire body. You can learn simple ways to control your own stress level and stay more relaxed, focused and happy.

Eat for Energy

Every meal is an opportunity to boost your health and energy. But what makes a healthy meal? It's simple. All you have to do is shift your thinking from "eat to get full" to eat to "feel good." A few simple guidelines will

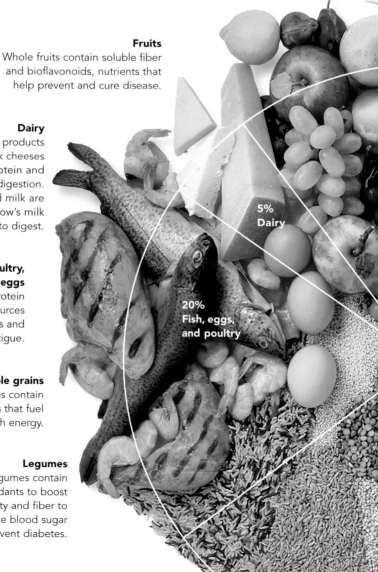

Fruits
Whole fruits contain soluble fiber and bioflavonoids, nutrients that help prevent and cure disease.

Dairy
Low-fat fermented dairy products like yogurt and skim milk cheeses provide calcium, protein and beneficial bacteria for digestion. Soy, rice and almond milk are good substitutes for cow's milk because they are easier to digest.

Fish, poultry, lean red meat and eggs
High quality protein from lean animal sources provides minerals and protein to prevent fatigue.

Whole grains
Whole grains contain carbohydrates that fuel your body with energy.

Legumes
Legumes contain antioxidants to boost immunity and fiber to balance blood sugar and prevent diabetes.

5% Dairy

20% Fish, eggs, and poultry

steer you towards the foods and the quantities that energize you and keep your weight under control. Your choice of what to eat is one of your most powerful tools for feeling your best.

What is soluble fiber?
Soluble fiber is found in vegetables, fruit and legumes. It removes toxins from the digestive system and slows down the absorption of carbohydrates (sugar) into the blood. This prevents the sugar highs and lows that can lead to diabetes, obesity and cardiovascular disease.

Vegetables
Vegetables contain minerals, vitamins and fuel for energy. They help reduce the risk of cancer and regulate body weight.

Beneficial oils
Olive oil is rich in antioxidants, which promote cell health and prevent inflammation and heart disease. Flax seed oil and other plant oils build and regenerate cell walls. Fish oil can prevent and treat many diseases of the heart, immune system, hormones and nervous system.

EATING

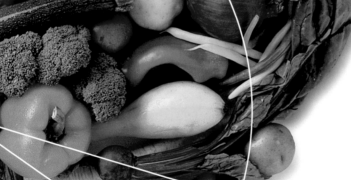

**40%
Fruits and vegetables**

**5%
Nuts and seeds**

**30%
Whole grains and legumes**

Nuts and seeds
Raw nuts and seeds are good sources of protein for energy and contain oils that benefit the brain and skin.

Drinking for Health

Water is life. It makes up 57% of your body and is essential for every chemical process that keeps you alive. Maintaining the right amount of water in your system keeps you energized by making your organs, blood

Water

We tell our patients to drink at least 8 glasses of water every day. In combination with other healthy drinks, consuming lots of water will keep your body hydrated, preventing fatigue and headaches. Keep a large bottle near your desk and in your car; make it easy to keep the water flowing. Clustered water, a new innovation, is water that has been treated with electricity. It can replenish your body's water more quickly than ordinary water.

Herbal, green and maté teas

Herbs have been made into hot drinks or tea for thousands of years. Tea is a quick, no-calorie alternative to juice or soft drinks. We recommend herbal teas, green tea and maté tea as healthy refreshing beverages. In addition to the benefits of the herbs themselves, tea is a great way to drink warm water, which is easier for your body to absorb than cold. Green tea contains powerful antioxidants that have been shown to promote health and fight cancer, as well as fat-burning nutrients.

100% fruit and vegetable juices

By juicing whole fruits and vegetables, you unlock a greater amount of nutrients and enzymes. All the minerals, antioxidants and vitamins are right there in the juice. Studies have shown that you will absorb more nutrients from the juice than you would from eating the whole fruit or vegetable. Try juicing carrot, apple, ginger, beet, tomato and parsley.

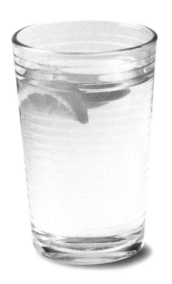
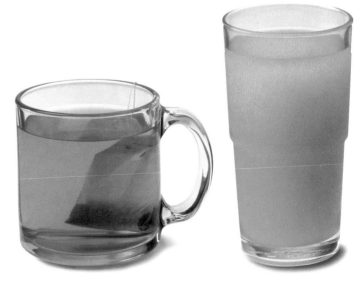

and cells do their jobs efficiently. Healthy drinks like these offer delicious options for getting vitamins and other nutrients to supplement the energy you get from healthy eating. Drink up!

Smoothies

Smoothies are made by combining healthy foods and nutritional supplements in a blender. You can use low-fat yogurt; fresh fruit juice; soy, rice or almond milk; whey protein powder; water and supplements. Blending in fresh or frozen banana slices or berries is a great way to add extra fruit. Watch out for commercial or unhealthy "smoothies" that contain sugar; these are just milkshakes in disguise.

Rehydration drinks

Drinks that contain sodium and other minerals are helpful for an active lifestyle. They replenish the minerals that are lost through stress and exercise. Athletes, business people and working mothers all find that taking rehydration drinks before and after physical activity prevents exhaustion and fatigue more effectively than drinking water alone.

Matay Slimming Energy Drink

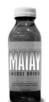

This energizing herbal beverage has the unique ability to wake up the mind without the nervousness and jitters often associated with coffee. It also has the added benefit of suppressing your appetite and encouraging weight loss. It contains the same amount of disease-fighting antioxidants as three servings of fruits and vegetables. To order, go to quixtar.com.

XS Energy Drink

This great-tasting, low-calorie energy drink is loaded with herbs like ginseng, astragalus and shizandra to increase energy and well-being. Many men and women report that XS helps them improve their energy for sports, work and daily activities. Athletes say that XS helps them keep up the intensity of their training programs. XS can be a great way to move towards a healthy lifestyle by replacing high fructose corn syrup (sugar) based soft drinks with a healthy, low-calorie alternative. To find out more, see page 70.

see page 70.

EATING

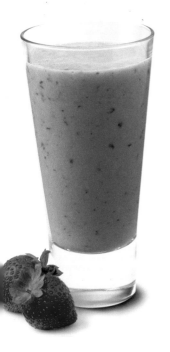

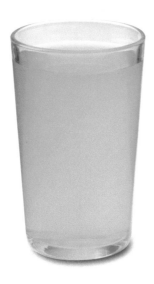

Energy-Draining Foods

No one chooses to eat high fat, high sugar, low fiber food because they think it is good for them. Most Americans consume food that is easy, fast and cheap. We encourage you to make your health your top priority and choose food for energy rather than convenience. Avoid these examples of the American "killer diet."

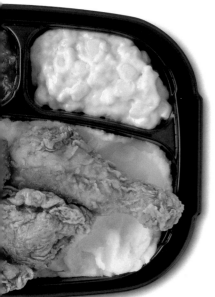

Refined sugar

Sugar can lead to obesity, diabetes, high blood pressure, heart disease, acne, mood disorders, Attention Deficit Disorder and cancer.
Found in: Most soft drinks, many breads, pastries, candy, cookies, "lean" meals

White flour

White flour has the carbohydrates of wheat, but it has been stripped of its nutritional value. It contains no fiber, no vitamin E and no B vitamins.
Found in: White bread, cookies, bagels, breakfast pastries

High saturated fats and oils

High saturated fat increases the risk for asthma, cardiovascular disease, Alzheimer's disease and prostate cancer.
Found in: Meat, dairy, deep-fried foods and snack foods

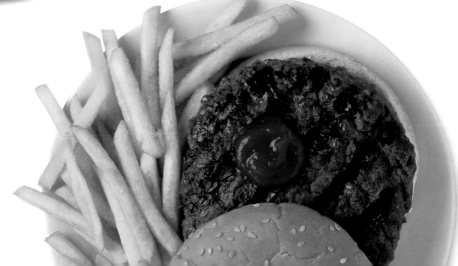

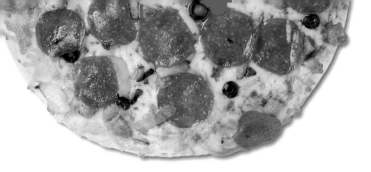

Dangerous drinking

Soda

The leading source of sugar in most peoples' diet is from soft drinks. A 12-oz can of soda contains 9 teaspoons of sugar! A 32-oz soda —typical large size soda at fast foods, malls or movie theaters— contains 24 teaspoons of sugar. Drinking this much sugar is believed to be the leading cause of diabetes, obesity, high blood pressure and heart disease.

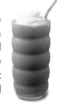

Over-sugared fruit drinks

"Flavored" fruit drinks are new ways of hiding unnecessary sugar in the form of high fructose corn syrup.

Milkshakes

Milkshakes are made from dairy and are high in saturated fat and sugar. A fruit smoothie has all the taste but none of the fat found in a milkshake.

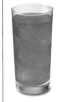

Alcohol

Four to five glasses of red wine a week is actually good for you. But over-consumption of beer, wine or spirits has a negative effect on health. Though it is a liquid, alcohol actually causes dehydration. It can also lead to diabetes, cirrhosis of the liver, birth defects, sleeping disorders, sexual dysfunction, cancer and heart problems.

EATING

Candy

Candy is nothing more than new and enticing ways to package sugar. Candy is like an empty box, covered with gift wrap and a big bow: looks good on the outside but there is nothing on the inside.

Refined and processed foods

Refined foods have been processed for appearance and convenience, but have lost most of their valuable nutrients. These foods are high in calories and low in fiber and cause obesity. Found in: "Instant" dinners, convenience foods, fast food and baked goods

Fatty meats

For the amount of protein it provides, fatty meat also contains more fat than most people can burn off. This can lead to weight gain, high blood pressure and cancer. Found in: Hamburgers, chicken wings, bacon, sausages, ribs, lamb, pork, hotdogs and other processed lunch meats

High sodium, salty foods

Excess salt can contribute to high blood pressure and dehydration. Even worse, salty foods tend to be snack foods (the number one food bought in America): high in sugar and low in nutrients. Found in: Fast food, snack foods, chips, salted pretzels, crackers

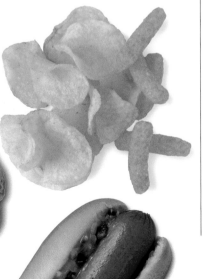

The Energized Plate

You can eat delicious, diverse meals and still lose weight. The key is eating the right amount of each type of food. Use your hand as a portion guide and leave the table full of energy, instead of just full.

You can measure healthy food portions with the parts of your hand. Use a fist for grains, a palm for meats, and thumbs for cheeses and oils.

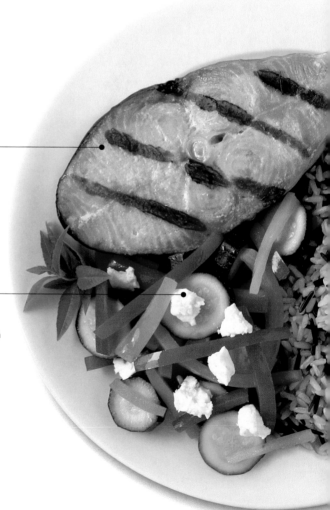

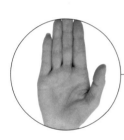

Fish, poultry, lean red meat
1 palm =
6-oz serving

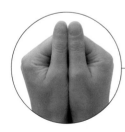

Hard cheeses (cheddar, parmesan) or feta
2 thumbs =
1-oz serving

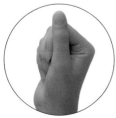

Olive, flax seed and plant oils
1 thumb =
1 tablespoon

Size matters

American portion sizes have increased drastically over the past 25 years. Today's restaurant servings, "super-size" meals and giant soft drinks contain much more fuel than your body can use.

Vegetables (and fruit)

Make sure your meals contain many servings of fruit and vegetables.

Whole grains, legumes, yogurt

1 fist = 1 cup

Nuts and seeds

1 handful =
1-oz serving

Less is more

Eating is a very visual experience. You will think you're eating larger portions if you serve your meals on a smaller plate...

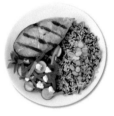

...versus the same serving portion placed on a larger dinner plate.

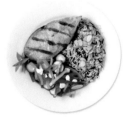

Healthy Cooking

How you prepare your food is almost as important as the food you cook. For example, steaming unlocks flavor and nutrients, while deep-frying adds saturated fat and empty calories you don't need. Try these healthy cooking methods and get the most out of the foods you eat.

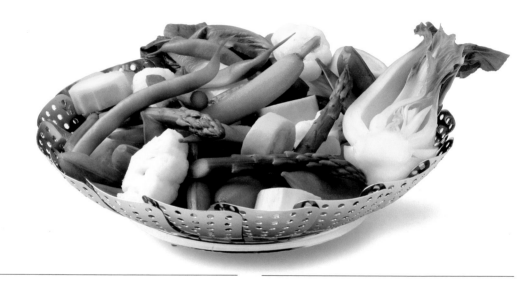

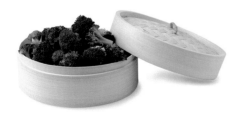

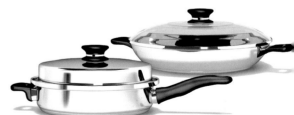

Steaming
Use a bamboo basket or a collapsible perforated steaming basket inside a saucepan with a ½ inch of water to steam your food. This is one of the best ways to keep flavors and nutrients intact.

Sautéing or stir-frying
Cooking small pieces or thin slices of vegetables or meat in a sauté pan or non-stick frying pan with a small amount of olive oil is a quick way to prepare a healthy meal in minutes.

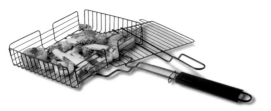

Grilling

Cooking over a hot flame or BBQ is a very healthy way to prepare meat because it drains away excess fat. You can marinate meat, fish and vegetables before cooking to add flavor.

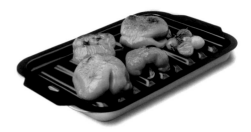

Broiling

Preparing food in the oven under a hot flame is a quick way to "grill" your food. Broiling gives a wonderful taste to meat, poultry, fish and vegetables.

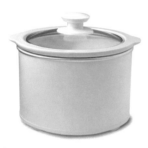

Slow cooking

Simmering at a low temperature over time retains nutrients and creates tender stews and beans. Because the pot is covered, the food will remain moist.

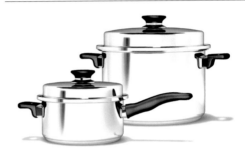

Low-moisture cooking

Cooking in a saucepan with a sealed lid locks in more natural flavors and nutrients while preserving color and texture. Brown your meats with no oil, then add a little liquid and cover to cook. Or place vegetables in a small amount of water, cover and steam until tender.

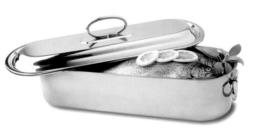

Poaching

Gently simmering with liquid in a fish poacher or saucepan is perfect for keeping cooked fish moist and flavorful. Poaching an egg in a saucepan of gently boiling water cooks it without the use of oil.

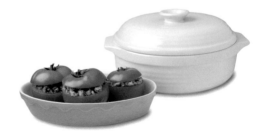

Baking and roasting

Cooking vegetables, casseroles or meats in the oven is an easy and flavorful way to prepare a main or side dish. Leaving the skins on vegetables helps retain nutrients and moisture.

Boost Your Food

Eating the right food is essential, but it is not enough. Because you are exposed to stress, environmental toxins and food that lacks key nutrients, we suggest that you take supplements. Just a couple of tablets

Pick the proper pill

There are thousands of different supplements and combinations available. So how do you choose? Start by thinking about you: How old are you? Are you male or female? Are you exposed to a great deal of stress? Do you have any medical conditions like high blood pressure or infections?

Look at the nutrients we describe on this page and identify the ones that address your needs. Start with a good daily multivitamin that gives you the main vitamins and minerals, and add any additional supplements that fit your individual situation.

VITAMINS & MINERALS

Vitamin A
Restores your immune system. Deficiency leaves the body open to bacterial and viral infections.

Vitamin D
Facilitates absorption of beneficial calcium into the body, regulates immune function.

Vitamin C
Helps improve immune function and prevent disease.

Vitamin B_3
Treats arthritis, diabetes and helps the body to produce energy.

Vitamin B_5
Pantothenic acid is the vitamin that helps the body cope with stress and allergies.

Vitamin B_6
Helps stabilize mood and mental state and improves ability to deal with stress.

Sodium
Prevents cramps and exhaustion.

Potassium
Important for nerve and muscle function.

Calcium
Helpful for high blood pressure, PMS, insomnia and restless leg syndrome.

Magnesium
Used to treat muscle spasms, diabetes, PMS, high blood pressure and kidney stones.

Chromium
Helps to stabilize blood sugar.

Zinc
Important in preventing diabetes and prostate swelling. Contributes to production of testosterone and growth hormone.

Manganese
Helps repair damaged discs and strengthen bone.

Selenium
An antioxidant, important for preventing cancer and enhancing immune function.

Iron
Carries oxygen in the blood to energize all the cells in the body.

Copper
Acts as an anti-inflammatory and antioxidant.

Folic acid
Prevents heart disease, cancer, anemia, depression, neural tube defects, restless leg syndrome and intestinal disorders.

a day of the right vitamins, minerals and herbs can boost your energy and prevent illness. Of the hundreds of nutrients available, these are the ones that we recommend for your new, energized life.

Which half are you in?
Studies show that almost half of the U.S. population are deficient in at least one of the following: Vitamin B_{12}, B_6, C, E, folic acid, iron or zinc.

Glutamine
Reduces stress and repairs muscle damage after exercise.

Arginine
Helps with immunity enhancement after exercise and trauma and contributes to wound healing and improved blood flow.

Taurine
Forces magnesium into cells, where it is needed for energy and performance. Also beneficial for people with cardiovascular problems.

5-HTP
Significantly reduces food cravings to promote weight loss.

BENEFICIAL PLANTS

Yerba maté
A tea made from the leaves of a South American tree, yerba maté helps energize the body and increases mental alertness. It contributes to weight loss by helping the body convert food into energy and by reducing appetite.

Ginseng
This plant root comes from Asia and has been used for centuries to enhance energy and performance. Doctors recommend it as a heart tonic, a stimulant and to improve sex drive. Studies show it can even improve symptoms of diabetes and reduce cholesterol. Patients with heart disease, stress, diabetes, poor digestion, weakness after illness and fatigue from aging report excellent results.

Maca
Originating in the South American mountains, this root increases the body's ability to handle physical and mental stress. Women have found it helps with PMS, menopause, low libido and fatigue. Men find it increases testosterone, sexual function, energy, stamina and the feeling of well-being.

Bioflavonoids
There are more than six thousand different bioflavonoid compounds found in fruits and vegetables. They work with the immune system and protect cells and body tissue from damage caused by toxins. This improves the health of vital organs like the heart, brain and liver. Look for bioflavonoids in multivitamin supplements.

ENERGY BOOSTERS

Caffeine
Caffeine (contained in coffee, green tea and XS Energy Drink) has many beneficial effects. It is a heart and brain stimulant, as well as a smooth muscle relaxant. Athletes take caffeine to enhance their performance. Caffeine has also been shown to increase the brain chemicals that improve concentration, focus and mood. A recent study showed that 90 mg of caffeine per day decreased the incidence of Alzheimer's and dementia. Consuming too much can make you feel anxious, so pay attention to your body and learn the amount that works for you.

Vitamin B_{12}
Vitamin B_{12} is the "energy" vitamin. People with fatigue often feel more energized by taking it daily. B_{12} is also helpful in bursitis, asthma, depression and anemia. Doses for B_{12} can be up to 1000 mg a day (several times the minimum recommended amount) without any adverse side effects. Depression can be an early sign of B_{12} deficiency.

EATING

Move Your Body

Your body is made to move. Every aspect of your health, from bone strength to blood flow, improves when you are physically active. So get moving! You don't need a gym, special clothing or expensive equipment to get the benefits of a body in motion. We can show you how to bring movement into your life quickly and easily. You will start at a level that is right for you. Then, as you feel more and more energized, you will build towards real and achievable goals. The best part is that you will start to feel an energy boost almost immediately!

BUILD ENDURANCE

Your body is designed to get up, go and then...keep going! This is called endurance and it is the first kind of fitness you will be building as you energize your life. We tell patients the great thing about endurance is that it is like interest at the bank: it builds on itself. Walking 10 minutes a day this week means your body will be ready for 20 minutes next week. It's natural. Endurance is the foundation that will let you stick with the movement program outlined in the Plan.

GAIN STRENGTH

Your muscles are incredibly smart: put them to work and they will adapt by becoming stronger. Strength is important for more than lifting heavier boxes: your muscles hold your entire body in alignment. So the more powerful your muscles are, the less likely you are to suffer back injury, joint pain or muscle strain. You can safely gain strength over time by following the Plan and letting your muscles do what they do naturally: grow stronger.

DEVELOP SKILLS

Once you build your healthy body, what will you use it for? By learning new patterns of movement like those found in ball sports, martial arts, snow sports or hiking you teach your body new ways to move. Even for beginners, there is incredible satisfaction in developing skill over time, and this will keep you inspired and moving. First work on endurance and strength, then after several months, pick up a sport or hiking.

Walk for life
Scientists estimate that, on average, each minute spent walking can extend your life by 1½ to 2 minutes!

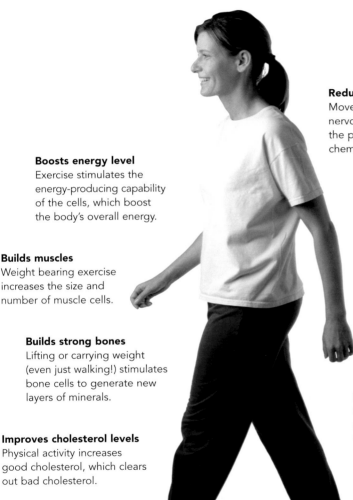

Reduces stress and anxiety
Movement regulates the nervous system and increases the production of "feel good" chemicals in the brain.

Boosts energy level
Exercise stimulates the energy-producing capability of the cells, which boost the body's overall energy.

Improves heart health
Movement improves heart function, circulation and blood clotting factors; stabilizes the heart rate; lowers blood pressure and decreases inflammation.

Builds muscles
Weight bearing exercise increases the size and number of muscle cells.

Stimulates weight loss
Exercise burns calories, melts abdominal fat and stimulates the body to burn fat all the time, even while we sleep.

Builds strong bones
Lifting or carrying weight (even just walking!) stimulates bone cells to generate new layers of minerals.

Helps prevent cancer
Physically active people have a lower incidence of cancer than those who are inactive.

Improves cholesterol levels
Physical activity increases good cholesterol, which clears out bad cholesterol.

Slows the aging process
Activity stimulates circulation, which removes toxins from the body. The buildup of toxins over time causes aging.

Ready, Set, Move

We often remind patients that if you want to get somewhere, start where you are right now. This applies to moving your body. Start by feeding your body the fuel it needs. Activate your muscles by warming them up. Then give your body enough time to recover between exercise sessions. You'll get maximum energy—and no injuries—by remembering to: "Fuel up, warm up and cool down."

GET FUELED UP

Give your blood all the water and nutrients it needs to feed your body's active muscles.

 3 hours before: Whey protein shake (recipe on page 44)

 1 hour before: 1 quart of rehydration drink

 15 minutes before: Only water

During exercise: Sip water—the more you sweat, the more you'll need.

BEFORE YOU EXERCISE

Warm up
Getting your body ready to move is child's play: Hop from foot to foot. Shake your arms. Swing your torso. Lift your knees. Remember jumping jacks? They are a perfect way to activate your body and loosen up. Warm up for 5 to 10 minutes and you'll be ready to go.

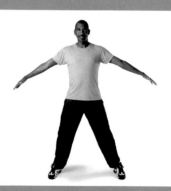

AFTER YOU EXERCISE

Stretch and cool down
Right after activity, don't just sit down—that's like slamming on the brakes. Instead, cool down gently by stretching and walking around slowly.

Eating after
Right after exercise, try a whey protein shake to replenish lost nutrients and help you bounce back.

Before your next session
Between exercise sessions, paying attention to recovery will give your body a chance to regenerate and prepare for more exercise. Help your body recover with rest, hydration, healthy food, sleep, stretching, hot baths and massage.

Why warm up?
A 5 to 10 minute routine—just enough to break a light sweat—prepares your body for activity and prevents muscle pulls, strains and soreness.

When to stop
Stop if you feel pain. Start slowly and build gradually. Make mental notes of your daily progress.

The right clothes
Wear light, breathable, comfortable clothing. Have a good water-shedding raincoat and pants so you can walk in all weather.

Safe salt
You lose salt (or sodium) when you sweat. A good way to replenish lost salt is with energy drinks that contain sodium and other minerals. Frequent urination at night after exercise is a sign of low sodium.

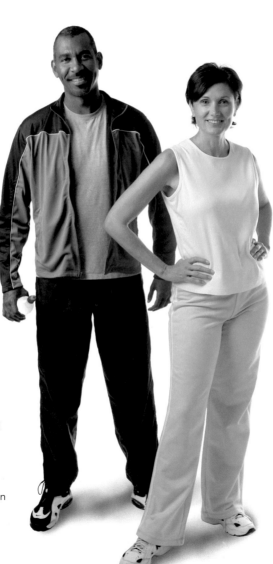

Good posture
Correct posture allows you to maximize efficiency and minimize injury. Keep your head, spine and hips in a straight line. Keep your shoulders back, in line with your ears.

Support bra
Women should be well supported during all activities. A support bra protects the back and

shoulders from fatigue and strain.

The right shoes
If your shoes give proper arch support, the feet, ankles, knees and hips will be properly aligned and cushioned. You will use less energy and feel less fatigued. Many exercise injuries start in the feet.

THE THREE KEYS

Put Motion in Your Life

Put your life in motion by putting motion in your life. It's easier than you think. Remember, your body was built to move! So why not give it a few more opportunities? Take the time you already spend on ordinary activities and put those minutes to work for you, boosting your energy. You will get huge health benefits by making even a few small changes in your daily routine. By moving throughout the day—every day— you will lose weight, reduce fatigue and improve your mood.

GET MOVING EVERY DAY

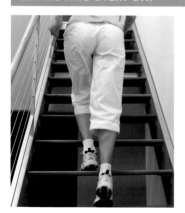

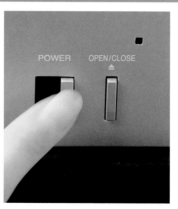

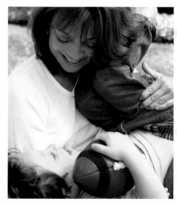

Take the stairs
Climbing stairs is fantastic exercise. Skip the elevator and walk: even a single flight up benefits your heart, lungs and legs.

Get off your chair
Don't use the remote to change the channel; get up and manually change it. Sit on an exercise ball instead of a chair to improve balance. Take a quick walk around the office while the computer is starting up.

Play with the kids
Kids have boundless energy. Actively playing with them gives you a natural boost. Try playing hide and seek or kicking and catching a ball. Ask your kids for suggestions. Who knows, maybe you'll even take up rollerblading!

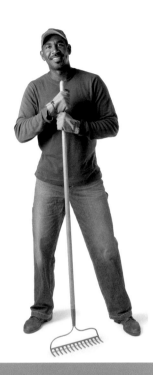

Walk away from obesity

A medical study of an Amish community showed that they were much healthier than typical Americans of the same age, with almost no obesity. The difference? Amish people walk one and a half to two times as much as most Americans. Walk on!

Backyard aerobics

Raking leaves, mowing the grass, weeding and trimming hedges offer diverse movements that can keep you as fit as an aerobics class.

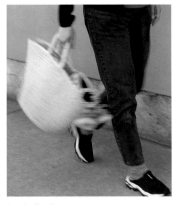

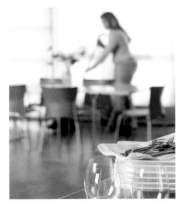

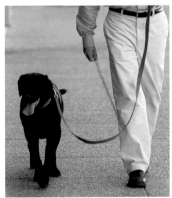

Park farther away

Instead of fighting over the spot closest to the store, deliberately park farther away from it. This integrates health and walking into every errand. Every step counts.

Clean the house

You have to do it anyway, so why not turn it into exercise? Do it quickly and with zest. Mopping, vacuuming, wiping windows—all of these tasks are opportunities to energize yourself with movement.

Walk the dog

Learn from your pet. Everyone knows dogs need to be walked, but we sometimes forget that we need to be walked, too!

Relax into Energy

Many people think of "relaxation" as simply the opposite of work, activity or stress—something to do on weekends. But it is much more. Relaxation is a recharging session for your body and mind. It balances body chemistry, lowers stress levels and improves oxygen flow. You can achieve a relaxed state in a variety of ways, by using visual, sound or body stimuli. We'll show you different techniques to try. When done every day, relaxation sends "calm down" signals to your entire nervous system. It promotes healing and enhances energy.

The foundation of relaxation

Because your brain responds to patterns, it is important to establish a pattern of relaxation. Do your relaxation training at the same time every day. Schedule a reasonable amount of time for your session so you don't feel rushed. And do it every day. Consistency and repetition will make your relaxation easier and more effective.

WHAT RELAXATION TYPE ARE YOU?

Vision-oriented

Some people have a natural talent for imagining how things look. They are able to envision machines, houses or sculptures before even putting down an image on paper. If this describes you, you'll find it easiest to relax through visual techniques. This might entail creating mental pictures of a relaxing situation, a changed circumstance or the body's healing energy.

Sound-oriented

For sound-oriented people, what they hear is their most important stimulus. Harsh noise like sirens and traffic make them stressed. Sound is also the key to helping them find relaxation. If this sounds like you, then listening to music, saying prayers, repeating affirmations and singing can all be used to help you balance your body and mind.

Body-oriented

Other people feel their most powerful sensations in their skin and entire body. If this is you, then relaxation techniques that involve touch, movement and breathing will be very powerful ways for you to balance your nervous system. Massage, chiropractic, acupuncture and yoga help body-dominant people eliminate stress.

Relaxation and happiness
Scientists using MRI brain scans have found that people who meditate using relaxation techniques activate the same part of the brain that is stimulated by feelings of happiness.

Reduces stress and anxiety
Relieving stress actually reduces the amount of the stress hormone cortisol in your blood. This hormone causes anxiety and depression.

Boosts immune function
The immune system works less effectively when under stress. Relaxation training can help cancer patients produce more of the blood cells that fight cancer.

Decreases blood pressure
Relaxation training opens up circulation, which improves blood flow and lowers blood pressure.

Regulates the digestive system
Anxiety and stress disturb digestion and aggravate every known disease of the stomach, intestines and colon.

Helps mental focus
A mind that is clear and refreshed from a relaxation session is capable of greater concentration.

Improves lung function
Stress constricts the lungs and reduces their capacity. Studies have shown that by using breathing methods and relaxation therapy, asthmatics can breathe easier and take less medication.

Balances menopause hormones
Stress suppresses production of the body's own natural hormones, which are already reduced by menopause. Learning to relax can help your body achieve hormonal balance.

RELAXING

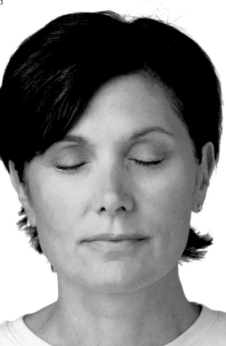

Relax Right Where You Are

We teach our patients that relaxation is not found on some far-off beach or distant vacation. It is as close as your breath, as your ears, as your closed eyes. And it is essential to realizing the full benefits of healthy food and movement. By taking a few moments a day for yourself, you can decrease your symptoms of stress: everything from anxiety to exhaustion. Like movement, relaxation is something you can bring into every day of your life, just by choosing to do so.

HOW TO RELAX MORE

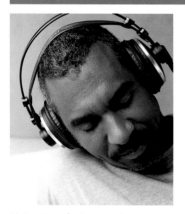 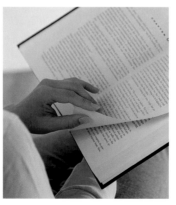 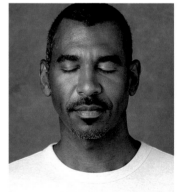

Listen to relaxing music
Research shows that soothing music puts the brain into a beneficial state.

Read a book you find inspiring
The thoughts of others can bring calm and feelings of well-being.

Remember to breathe
Take a deep breath, reflect and count to 10.

SYMPTOMS OF STRESS

Anxiety
Fearful or nervous thoughts about the past and future.

Night sweats
Spontaneous sweating in the middle of the night.

Post-exercise fatigue
After exercising, you feel run down instead of relaxed and energized.

Allergy symptoms
Increase in sneezing, congestion and facial puffiness from hay fever and other allergies.

Mood problems
Sudden changes in mood or unexplained sadness, fear or anger.

Heart palpitations
Feeling the heart flutter or beat in the chest.

Paranoia
Unreasonable fear of people or situations.

Fatigue
Feeling tired on waking from sleep and throughout the day.

Muscle and joint aches
Body aches after slight exertion.

Sleeplessness
Inability to fall asleep or waking in the middle of the night.

Depression
Lack of enthusiasm for family, work and friends.

Memory lapses
Difficulty or inability to recall recent events.

Concentration problems
Difficulty focusing and staying focused on a task.

Stress is real
MRI brain scans show that stress and emotional pain activate the same parts of the brain as physical pain. Take stress as seriously as you would an injury and reduce it by relaxing every day.

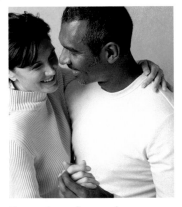

Dance, have fun or play a game
Fun brings laughter and releases tension.

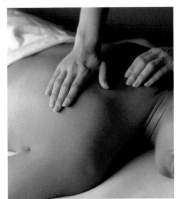

Get a massage or take a sauna
Being touched or warmed brings a feeling of safety and calm.

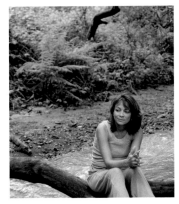

Take a walk or watch a sunset
Even a short journey into the beauty of nature brings calm to the mind and body.

Sleep for Health

A night of good sleep is just as important to optimal health and energy as food and exercise. Lack of sleep makes you feel tired, but it also affects hormone levels, decreases mental clarity and has negative effects on your overall health. While some people sleep more easily than others, anyone can learn good sleep habits.

How much is enough sleep?
Researchers have found humans need a minimum of 8 hours of sleep a night. Depending on your age, you may need as much as 12 hours a night. Most Americans operate at a "sleep deficit," getting 7 hours or less sleep each night.

What are sleep cycles?
A good night's sleep includes up to 4 sleep cycles. Each cycle is a series of different brain states that all work together to let the brain and body regenerate. To get the full benefit of sleep, each cycle must be completed. This is why sleep that is interrupted by insomnia or noise is less restful than a night of continuous sleep.

LOSING SLEEP

Insomnia
Insomnia is the inability to get to sleep or to sleep through the night. It can cause health problems and is an epidemic among American adult women, with 25% saying they have insomnia.

Sleep-onset insomnia
Difficulty falling asleep is often accompanied by thoughts that "just won't stop" when it is time for bed. As a result, sleep does not begin until the early morning hours. In the morning, sufferers of sleep-onset insomnia are still in the middle of their sleep process, so they wake up feeling groggy and disoriented.

Sleep-maintenance insomnia
Some people wake in the middle of the night, after several hours of sleep, no longer feeling tired. It is then difficult to fall asleep again. Sleep is not established and maintained for an entire night, so the full benefits are not obtained.

Consequences of sleep shortage
Decreased physical performance, strength and speed

Difficulty learning new tasks

Diminished brain performance

Less alertness

Bad mood and negative attitude

Obesity

Diabetes

Cardiovascular disease

Stress

Low testosterone

Decline in immunity

Chronic fatigue

Joint problems

Insomnia

Decreased sexual desire

Depression

Osteoporosis

SLEEP BENEFITS

Sleep away sickness
People with chronic sleep problems have more than twice as many sick days as good sleepers.

Balances mood
Sleep balances the production of brain chemicals that create a sense of well-being. Sleep leaves you physically and mentally refreshed.

Controls blood sugar
Sleep helps regulate your blood sugar level, improving your energy and preventing diabetes.

Improves immune function
White blood cells are more active against viruses and bacteria when you are rested.

Enhances learning
Trying a new task and then sleeping speeds up how quickly you learn it.

Increases energy
Sleep leaves you physically and mentally refreshed.

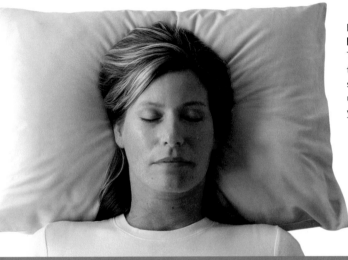

RELAXING

HOW TO SLEEP BETTER

Before going to bed
Don't eat for 4 hours before bedtime.

Drink chamomile tea, other herbal tea or warm milk.

Have a hot bath. Listen to relaxing music or read something relaxing.

Take a capsule of the herb valerian. Use the extract (0.8% valerenic acid) and take 150 to 300 mg.

Try not to fall asleep on the sofa or in front of the TV.

While you're in bed
Go to bed at the same time every night and get up at the same time every morning.

Don't use your bed for work.

Sleep in a quiet, dark room: use curtains or an eye mask to block light, earplugs to block noise.

Try using breathing techniques and relaxation methods in bed before sleeping.

If you wake up in the middle of the night
Get out of bed and read for 30 minutes.

Do breath training described on page 57.

Do not watch TV.

Try a brief cold shower or a lukewarm bath for 30 minutes.

If your mind is working on problem solving, write the problems down and decide to deal with them in the morning.

Welcome to the Plan: your roadmap to a more energized life. For the next three weeks, the Plan will help you choose what to eat, teach you ways to get your body moving and show you how to relax your body and mind. By using these three

The Three-Week Plan

powerful keys, you will actually see yourself change. And you will feel better long before the three weeks are over. Though 21 days is a short time, we know from experience that it is enough for you to reinvent yourself, break old habits and build a foundation for an energized life. The Plan is your coach. If at any time you feel unsure of what to eat or do, just come back to the Plan. It will help you make the choices that help you look and feel your best.

Week 1: Eat for energy

For the first week of your journey, you will focus on cleansing your body and stepping out of your old patterns. You can do this! Simple foods, easy movements and basic relaxation will form the foundation for the rest of the Plan. You'll be feeling results before the week is over.

Week 2: Move forward

Week 2 is all about bridging the gap between breaking old habits and creating healthy new ones. You'll eat more protein this week as you step up your movement program and add new relaxation tools. Expect to see some weight loss and feel much more energized.

Week 3: Plan for life

As you arrive at Week 3, you will be looking and feeling healthier, so you won't want to stop now. You'll round out your food options with even more variety, and you'll find a movement program that suits you for the long term. This week starts you on your way to a lifetime of energy and health.

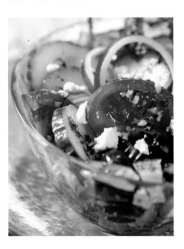

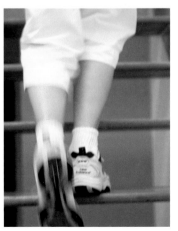

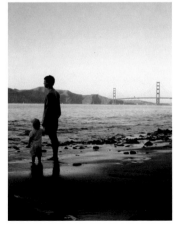

WEEK 1

WEEK 2

WEEK 3

Week 1: Eat for Energy

What to expect
You may feel light-headed as your body adapts to high-energy, easy-to-digest foods. Notice the changes in your body as you drop old habits, and expect an energy surge around Days 5 to 7.

For the first week of the Plan, the goal is cleansing your body. The most noticeable change will be the food you eat. It will be a bit more limited this week than later in the Plan. You'll also embark on a light movement program to get your body in action and you'll learn easy relaxation techniques to fight stress. Expect to lose some weight and to feel a surge of confidence from seeing immediate, positive results.

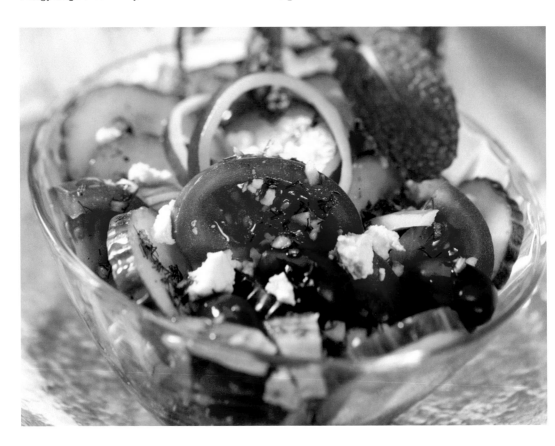

Wake-up

Drink 8-oz hot lemon water (recipe, page 44)

Begin core stability exercises (page 47)

Do visualization training (page 49)

Morning

Eat fruit and/or drink 8-oz protein shake or smoothie (recipe, page 44)
Eat 2-4 rice cakes
Consume 10-oz Matay Slimming Energy Drink
Take vitamin supplements (page 43)

Matay Slimming Energy Drink is made with yerba maté and other herbs, like maca, that stimulate weight loss and energize your body. Taken three times a day, you will see results within the first week. To order, go to quixtar.com.

Mid-morning

Eat fruit and/or drink 8-oz protein shake or smoothie
Consume 10-oz Matay Slimming Energy Drink

Noon

Eat salad and vegetable-based soup (recipe, page 44)
OR eat 1 cup rice or legumes or 1 baked yam with steamed vegetables (recipe, page 44)
Consume 10-oz Matay Slimming Energy Drink

Afternoon

Eat fruit and/or drink 8-oz protein shake or smoothie
Eat 2-4 rice cakes

Warm up (jump up and down 5 times) and walk 10 minutes

Schedule your walk at the same time every day. Make it as important as showing up for work on time.

Evening

Eat salad and vegetable-based soup
OR eat 1 cup rice or legumes or 1 baked yam with steamed vegetables

Eat a lighter meal or a smaller portion for dinner because your metabolism slows down in the evening.

Before sleep

Drink 8-oz hot herbal tea

Do resting pose (page 48) and go to sleep

WEEK 1

_{WEEK} **1** | Daily Food Choices

Beverages **Many servings**		Lemon water; purified water; herbal, green and maté teas	Avoid: Soda and diet sodas, sweetened juices and drinks, alcohol; high-calorie coffee drinks
Fruit **Many servings**		Eat any fruit. To ease digestion, eat only one kind at a time. High in soluble fiber: apples, plums and pears	
Vegetables **Many servings**	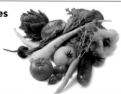	Eat a variety of vegetables in any combination. High in soluble fiber: beets, carrots, broccoli	Avoid: Corn
Grains **2 cups**		Rice: brown, basmati, jasmine, wild rice; rice cakes Grains: quinoa, millet, amaranth	Avoid: White rice, flour, wheat, barley, breakfast cereals and any products containing these ingredients (for example, white or wheat bread, pasta)
Legumes **2 cups**		Mung beans, bean sprouts, tofu, soybeans, red lentils, miso One cup of mung beans is full of protein and soluble fiber.	Avoid: All other legumes this week

Fats and oils **Up to** **2 tablespoons**	Extra virgin olive oil only Extra virgin olive oil is natural and high in cancer-fighting antioxidant vitamins. Use it for cooking, on salads and for seasoning.	Avoid: All others fats and oils this week
Condiments **As needed**	Vegetable, seasoned or sea salt; apple cider, balsamic and rice vinegars; wheat-free tamari; all spices; miso	Avoid: Ketchup, mayonnaise, BBQ sauce, relish, mustard, salad dressing, packaged oil- or liquid-based seasoning (for example,chutney, Chinese sauces with MSG)
Supplements For more information on supplements, see page 70.	Whey protein powder (2 servings) Multivitamin (one daily serving) Vitamin C (500 mg) Matay Slimming Energy Drink (three 10-oz servings)	

Shopping list

Fresh vegetables

Fresh fruit

Lemons

Brown, basmati or wild rice

Quinoa, millet or amaranth

Mung or soy beans or red lentils

Tofu

Rice cakes

Soy or rice milk

Herbal, green or maté tea

Apple cider, balsamic or rice vinegar

Wheat-free tamari

Miso

Extra virgin olive oil

Vegetable or sea salt

Whey protein powder

Multivitamins and vitamin C

Other foods to avoid this week

No meats, poultry, fish, eggs

No dairy: butter, ice cream, yogurt (substitute soy or rice milk for cow's milk)

No nuts and seeds

No chocolate

No refined sugar, honey, molasses

No jams

No foods with preservatives or food coloring

No packaged, processed or canned food

No fast food

WEEK 1

1 WEEK | Recipes

DAILY

Lemon Water

Wash one organic lemon and cut in half. Squeeze one half of the lemon into a half gallon of water. Add the squeezed lemon and the remaining half to the water. Drink hot or cold.

BREAKFAST & SNACKS

Breakfast Smoothie

1 cup fruit (fresh or frozen peeled banana or berries, or freshly squeezed orange juice)
2 tbsp whey protein powder
1 cup plain or vanilla soy milk
1 tsp ground flax seed or cinnamon, optional

In a blender add all of the ingredients. Cover and blend until smooth. Serves 1.

Quick Protein Shake

1 cup soy milk or fresh fruit juice
2 tbsp whey protein powder

Pour the soy milk or juice into a blender and add the protein powder. Cover and blend until smooth. Serves 1.

LUNCH & DINNER

Vegetable Soup

4 cups vegetable stock
½ cup celery, chopped
2 carrots, peeled and sliced
1 tomato, cored and diced
½ cup green beans, minced
1 red or Yukon Gold potato, diced
Minced fresh herbs to taste
    (basil, oregano, parsley or dill)
Salt and pepper to taste

Bring the stock to a simmer in a large saucepan. Add the vegetables (add other vegetables as you like). Simmer for 20 minutes, until the vegetables are tender. Season with fresh herbs, salt and pepper. Serves 4.

Steamed Vegetables

2 pounds assorted vegetables (cauliflower, broccoli, bok choy, brussels sprouts, zucchini, snow peas, green beans, carrots)

Wash vegetables and cut into bite-sized pieces. Place vegetables in the top of a steamer (or in a covered saucepan) with 1 inch of water in the bottom. Put the vegetables that require the longest cooking time at the bottom with the softer ones on top. Heat until the water boils, then turn down the heat and cook for 5 to 15 minutes, until the vegetables are tender, but firm. Drain (if necessary) and serve with brown or basmati rice. Serves 4.

Hearty Vegetable Salad

4 to 6 cups mixed baby greens, washed
1 to 2 cups broccoli, lightly steamed and chopped
1 carrot, peeled and sliced
1 celery stalk, sliced
½ each red and yellow pepper, chopped
½ cucumber, sliced
¼ cup green onions, chopped
1 cup whole cherry tomatoes
1 avocado, sliced
1 cup whole snow peas, lightly steamed
¼ cup dried cranberries or organic blueberries

Toss the mixed baby greens and vegetables in a salad bowl. Sprinkle with dried cranberries or organic blueberries. Serve with or without the Ginger Orange Dressing. Serves 4 to 6.

Ginger Orange Dressing

1 clove garlic
1 tsp dried Italian herb blend
2 tsp raw ginger, grated
¼ to ½ cup extra virgin olive oil
¼ cup rice or apple cider vinegar
½ seedless orange, peeled (with white pith removed)

In a blender place all of the ingredients. Cover and blend until smooth. Serves 4 to 6.

For more tasty recipes, please visit www.energizeyourlife.com.

Roasted Root Vegetables

1 to 2 potatoes or yams
2 large carrots
1 or 2 parsnips
1 rutabaga
1 to 2 red or yellow beets
1 onion, peeled and cut
   into ¼-inch pieces
1 head garlic, separated into
   cloves and peeled
1 to 2 tbsp extra virgin olive oil
Salt, herbs (rosemary and thyme)
   and balsamic vinegar to taste

Preheat oven to 400 degrees. Peel and chop the vegetables into 1-inch pieces. Place root vegetables, onion and garlic in a large bowl and toss with olive oil and salt. Pour the vegetables into a large roasting pan (or cookie sheet with edges), keeping the vegetables in a single layer. Roast 35 to 45 minutes, turning once or twice during this time, until the vegetables are tender and slightly browned. Add salt, herbs and balsamic vinegar to taste. Serves 4 to 6.

Variation: Use this basic roasting technique for a single type of root vegetables (for example, roast only potatoes with dried herbs, salt and pepper to taste).

DESSERT

Kheir Rice Pudding

2 cups water
1 cardamom pod
1 2-inch cinnamon stick
2 or 3 black peppercorns
½ cup raisins
¼ cup cashews
1 cup white basmati rice
2⅛ cup soy milk, heated

In a saucepan bring 2 cups of water to a boil. Add the spices, raisins, cashews and rice. Reduce heat and simmer, covered, for 15 to 20 minutes, until the water is absorbed. Add 2 cups of heated soy milk and cook on low heat, uncovered, for 30 to 40 minutes. Stir a few times to keep the rice from sticking to the bottom. Add ⅛ cup of soy milk to thin, if needed. Sprinkle with cinnamon, if desired.

Why no wheat?

Although whole wheat has many nutrients, wheat often causes allergic reactions. It slows down the rate at which the body burns calories and so can contribute to weight gain. Eating a lot of wheat has been linked to arthritis, headaches, fatigue, sleepiness and diarrhea. We have found that by cutting wheat out of their diets, our patients lose weight, have more energy and show less facial puffiness. Instead of wheat-based products, go to a health food store and look for:

- Whole rye or rice-based breads

- Buckwheat (soba), soy or thread bean noodles

- Millet or quinoa breakfast cereal

- Buckwheat pancakes

WEEK 1

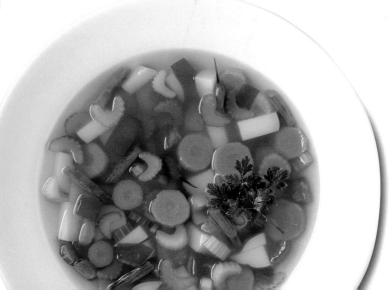

WEEK 1 | Get Moving

Get up and get moving
To avoid missing a single day, schedule your movement minutes first thing in the morning. This way, you won't find that, "Oops!" the entire day has gone by without being active. And you'll feel the benefits even sooner.

Humans were designed by nature to move an equivalent of walking six to nine miles a day. Daily walking, the most basic form of exercise, is great for your health. It keeps blood sugar down, burns abdominal fat and keeps your mood positive. This week, we "reintroduce" you to walking, as well as to a core stability exercise. Together, these two simple activities are the foundation that will let you safely add more movement to your life in the weeks ahead.

WALKING	10 MINUTES

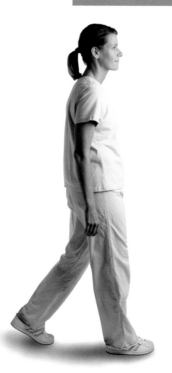

Walking is so good for you, it's worth doing even more than the Plan recommends. And it's easy to bring into your life. You don't have to join a gym, just get out the door and go. Walk around the office, walk to the store and walk up stairs.

Your "core" is the system of abdominal muscles that supports your internal organs and your back. Strengthening it reduces back pain, improves posture and prevents injuries that can result from simple tasks like reaching up to a high shelf and turning over in bed. Weakness of these muscles can come from poor posture and long hours of sitting at a desk or in front of the TV.

Step 1

1. Lie on your back with knees bent, feet flat on the floor.

2. Press your lower back to the floor so there is not enough room to put your fingers between your spine and the floor.

3. Place your hands on your stomach and feel the abdominal muscles contract.

4. Hold your lower back in this position against the floor throughout the entire core stability exercise.

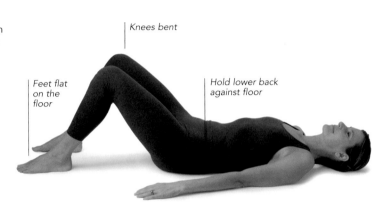

Knees bent

Feet flat on the floor

Hold lower back against floor

Step 2

1. Lift your right knee up and down 5 times, keeping the foot 1 inch off the ground and holding the lower back to the floor.

2. Repeat with the left knee. Do this exercise while slowly counting to 4. Slowly inhale while lifting the foot up. Slowly exhale while bringing the foot down to a count of 4, keeping the foot 1 inch off the ground.

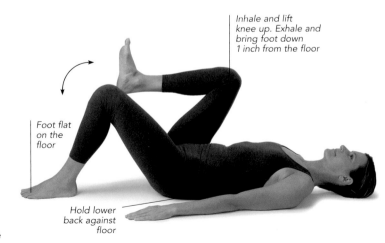

Inhale and lift knee up. Exhale and bring foot down 1 inch from the floor

Foot flat on the floor

Hold lower back against floor

WEEK 1

For more physical activities, please visit www.energizeyourlife.com.

WEEK 1 | Begin to Relax

Make an appointment
Our culture is so action-oriented that it can be hard to make time for relaxation. Take charge by picking a time of day that works for you and commit to the same 10-minute slot every day. Many people find that relaxing right before dinner works well.

This week, you will experience the powerful connection between your body and your mind. This is the key to making the changes you want to make in your life. Our internal image of ourselves represents everything meaningful in our life: our hopes, our intentions and our goals. Whether you are trying to change your body, your relationships or your work life, you can help the process by relaxing and visualizing.

RESTING POSE   5 MINUTES

Resting Pose is a simple but surprisingly powerful technique. It may look like "just lying there" but in fact the position sends signals to your entire body, telling it to relax, slow down and recharge.

1. Lie flat on your back with your eyes closed, your arms and legs slightly apart, palms facing up.

2. Focus on your breath, which should be long, slow and deep.

3. Focus on your feet and relax them.

4. Focus and relax in the same way on the legs, the abdomen, the hands, the arms, the chest, the neck, the face and finally the mouth.

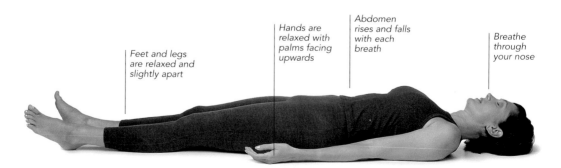

Feet and legs are relaxed and slightly apart

Hands are relaxed with palms facing upwards

Abdomen rises and falls with each breath

Breathe through your nose

This technique is especially good for body-oriented people.

Visualization is simply deciding on an image to "see" in your mind's eye and then picturing it. You imagine things all the time without thinking about it. Images of yourself or your expectations are always going through your mind. These unconscious pictures can sometimes be negative. The powerful thing about visualization is that you decide what to imagine and so you make it a positive experience.

2. Breathe slowly in and out three times, with eyes closed. Relax deeper and deeper each time you exhale. After these exhalations, repeat the image of what you want to change and then change the picture to match the way you would like things to be.

1. Breathe slowly in and out three times, with eyes closed. Relax deeper and deeper each time you exhale. After these exhalations, visualize an image of yourself or an aspect of your life that you want to change (for example, being overweight, having poor memory, fighting with your spouse, poor job performance).

3. Breathe slowly in and out three times, with eyes closed. Relax deeper and deeper each time you exhale. After these exhalations, visualize the new image with no trace of the old image remaining. Keep that image with you.

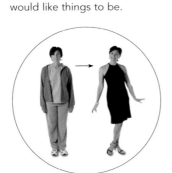

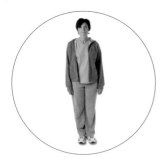

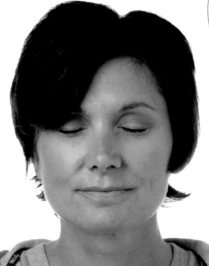

This technique is especially good for vision-oriented people.

For more relaxation techniques, please visit www.enerergizeyourlife.com

WEEK 1

Week 2: Move Forward

As you enter Week 2 of the Plan, you're feeling more energy than usual and it is likely you have lost some weight. This week builds on your momentum towards higher energy and greater weight loss by stepping up your level of physical activity. You will eat more protein in the form of eggs, fish, poultry and nuts. A new relaxation technique will energize and de-stress you. As you reach the Plan's halfway point at midweek, there will be no stopping you.

What to expect:
Having cleansed your body in Week 1, you can now start to add high-protein food back into your diet. You'll eat more than last week, and your emphasis will be on bringing more movement into your daily life.

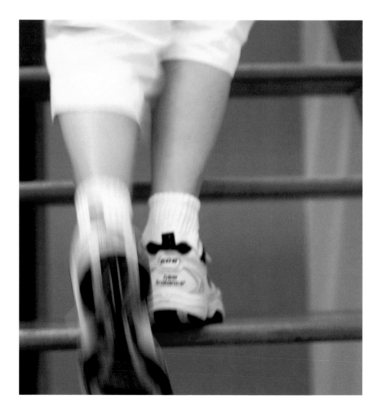

Wake-up

Drink 8-oz hot lemon water (recipe, page 44)

Begin core stability exercises (page 56)

Do breath training (page 57)

Hot lemon water relaxes the digestive system and energizes blood circulation.

Morning

Eat fruit and/or drink 8-oz protein shake or smoothie (recipe, page 44)
OR eat 1-2 poached eggs with rye bread (recipe, page 54)
Eat 2-4 rice cakes
Consume 10-oz Matay Slimming Energy Drink
Take vitamin supplements (page 53)

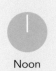

Mid-morning

Eat fruit and/or drink 8-oz protein shake or smoothie
Consume 10-oz Matay Slimming Energy Drink

Noon

Eat one 6-oz serving of poultry with salad and vegetable-based soup (recipe, page 44)
OR eat 1 cup rice or 1 baked yam or legumes with steamed vegetables (recipe, page 44)
Consume 10-oz Matay Slimming Energy Drink

Afternoon

Eat fruit and/or drink 8-oz protein shake or smoothie
Eat 2-4 rice cakes

Warm up (jump up and down 5 times) and walk 20 minutes

Evening

Eat salad and vegetable-based soup
OR eat 1 cup rice or 1 baked yam or legumes with steamed vegetables

Before sleep

Drink 8-oz hot herbal tea

Do resting pose (page 48) or breath training (page 57) and go to sleep

WEEK 2

WEEK 2 | Daily Food Choices

Items in red are new foods this week.

Beverages
Many servings

Lemon water; purified water; herbal, green and maté teas

Avoid:
Soda and diet sodas, sweetened juices and drinks, alcohol; high-calorie coffee drinks

---

Fruit
Many servings

Eat any fruit. To ease digestion, eat only one kind at a time.

Blueberries have a high soluble fiber content and are rich in antioxidants.

Vegetables
Many servings

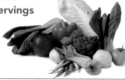

Eat a variety of vegetables in any combination.

High in soluble fiber:
green beans, zucchini, acorn squash

Grains
2 cups

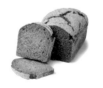

Rice: brown, basmati, jasmine, wild rice; rice cakes; rice-based breads
Grains: quinoa, millet, amaranth, teff, kasha (roasted buckwheat), whole rye bread (2 slices)

Avoid:
White rice, flour, wheat, barley, breakfast cereals and any products containing these ingredients (for example, white or wheat bread, pasta)

Legumes
2 cups

Mung beans, bean sprouts, tofu, soybeans, lentils, miso, chick peas, adzuki beans, pinto beans, kidney beans, split peas, black-eyed peas, white beans, soy milk

Avoid:
Any legume that causes intestinal discomfort. If using canned beans, drain and rinse them well before using.

Fats and oils
Up to
2 tablespoons

Extra virgin olive oil only

Avoid:
Margarine, butter, hydrogenated fats and other oils

Shop organic
Buy organic produce when possible—it is higher in nutrients and will taste better.

53

Condiments **As needed**	Vegetable, seasoned or sea salt; apple cider, balsamic and rice vinegars; wheat-free tamari; all spices; miso; low-calorie mayonnaise; mustard	Avoid: MSG, regular mayonnaise, artificial flavors, preservatives, sugary relishes, bottled salad dressings
Nuts and seeds **1-oz serving**	Raw nuts: almond, pecan, walnut, hazelnut, Brazil, cashew, pine nuts, macadamia, pistachio Raw seeds: sunflower, sesame, poppy, pumpkin	Avoid: Peanuts and all nuts that are roasted, dry-roasted, canned or salted
Poultry and fish **6-oz serving** **Eggs** **2 eggs = 1 serving**	Poultry: turkey, chicken, goose, guinea fowl, pheasant, duck Fish: crab, shrimp, lobster, halibut, herring, mackerel, salmon, sardines To save time, use canned fish.	Avoid: Farmed fish, fish high in mercury (swordfish, tuna)
Supplements For more information on supplements, see page 70.	Whey protein powder (2 servings) Multivitamin (one daily serving) Vitamin C (500 mg) Matay Slimming Energy Drink (three 10-oz servings)	

Shopping List

Fresh fruit, lemons

Fresh vegetables

Brown, basmati or wild rice

Teff or kasha

Whole rye or rice-based breads

Adzuki, pinto, mung, kidney, white or soy beans; chick, black-eyed or split peas; lentils

Tofu

Rice cakes

Soy, rice or almond milk

Nuts and seeds

Fish or poultry

Eggs (preferably free range)

Herbal, green or maté tea

Other foods to avoid this week

No red meat

No dairy (replace with soy, rice or almond milk)

No chocolate, sugar, honey, jams, molasses, foods with preservatives or food coloring

No packaged, processed or fast foods

WEEK 2 | Recipes

BREAKFAST

Banana Breakfast Blender

1 fresh or frozen peeled banana
2 tbsp whey protein powder
1 cup soy milk

In a blender add the banana and whey protein powder. Pour in the soy mile. Cover and blend until smooth. Serves 1.

Nutty Cinnamon Apple Oatmeal

1 cup unsweetened apple juice
½ cup water
½ tsp ground cinnamon
⅛ tsp salt
¾ cup rolled oats
⅓ cup soy milk
2 tbsp walnuts, chopped

Combine the apple juice, water, cinnamon and salt in a small saucepan and bring to a boil. Stir in rolled oats. Reduce heat and cook for 5 minutes, stirring occasionally. Heat the soy milk. Serve the oatmeal in bowls and pour on the hot soy milk. Sprinkle with walnuts. Serves 2.

Poached Eggs with Rye Bread

2 quarts water
1 tsp vinegar
2 tsp salt
4 large fresh eggs

Place water, vinegar and salt in a saucepan and bring to a boil. Crack the eggs into individual bowls so that you can reduce heat to simmer and gently slide the eggs into the boiling water. Turn off heat and cover the saucepan. Let the eggs poach with the residual heat for 3 to 3½ minutes. Remove the eggs with a slotted spoon and drain any excess water. Serve with 2 to 4 slices of toasted whole rye bread. Serves 2.

LUNCH & DINNER

Brown Rice Carrot Nut Loaf

1 cup mixed brown rice and wild rice
2 cups water
1 vegetarian bouillon cube
½ onion, chopped
1 large carrot, grated
½s cup raw walnuts, chopped
1 egg, beaten
Parmesan cheese, grated

Combine rices, water and bouillon cube in a saucepan and bring to a boil. Cook the rice for 45 minutes. Mix in the onion, carrot, walnuts and egg. Pour into baking dish. Bake at 350 degrees for 40 minutes. Top with grated parmesan cheese. Serves 4 to 6.

Poached Salmon

2 to 4 6-oz salmon fillets
1 carrot, sliced
1 small onion, sliced
1 stalk celery, sliced
2 slices lemon
Small bunch of parsley
1 bay leaf
1 to 3 cups vegetable stock or water
Salt to taste
Juice of half a lemon

In a saucepan place the carrot, onion, celery, lemon slices, parsley and bay leaves. Add the salmon (skin side down), stock or water to cover, salt to taste and the lemon juice. Bring to a boil, uncovered. Adjust heat to simmer, cover with lid and cook for 5 minutes. Turn off the heat and leave fish undisturbed for 10 minutes, until salmon is perfectly done. Remove fish to a serving platter. Serve either hot or cold. Eat with steamed rice and vegetables. Serves 2 to 4.

For more tasty recipes, please visit www.energizeyourlife.com.

Rainbow Spinach Salad

4 to 6 cups spinach, washed
½ cup red onion, thinly sliced
½ each red, orange and yellow
  peppers, thinly sliced
½ cup mandarin orange slices or
  green grapes
3 tbsp dried cranberries
¼ cup chopped walnuts or
  slivered almonds
¼ cup crumbled goat or soy feta
  or grated Parmesan cheese

Place the washed spinach in a
large salad bowl. Add onion,
peppers, fruit, nuts and cheese.
Add Berry Dressing to taste
and toss the salad lightly to coat.
Serves 4 to 6.

Berry Dressing

¼ cup extra virgin olive oil
½ cup frozen berries
¼ cup apple cider vinegar

In a blender add all of the
ingredients. Cover and blend
until smooth. Makes ¾ cup.

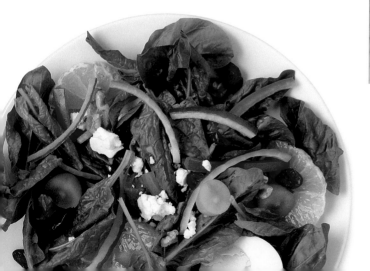

SNACK

Hummus

1 cup garbanzo beans
⅓ cup tahini or sesame butter
1 clove of garlic, chopped
⅓ cup parsley, chopped
Juice of 1 lemon
1 tsp cumin
Salt to taste
⅛ tsp pepper
1 tbsp extra virgin olive oil

In a food processor combine
all of the ingredients and purée.
Thin with more olive oil, lemon
juice or water, if needed. Use
as a dip for carrots, celery and
other vegetable slices or as a
sandwich spread on rye bread.
Serves 4 to 6.

Suggested cooking times for 1 cup of rice or grains

Water (cups)	Cooking time	Yield (cups)
Basmati rice		
1¾	20 min	3
Brown rice		
2	45 min	3
Wild rice		
2	50 min	2¾
Amaranth		
2½	20 min	2½
Kasha		
2	2 min	2½
Millet		
3	40 min	3½
Pearled barley		
2	55 min	3
Quinoa		
2	20 min	2½
Quinoa flakes		
2	5 min	2½
Rolled oats		
2	15 min	2½
Steel-cut oats		
2	25 min	2½
Whole oats		
3	60 min	3½

WEEK 2

WEEK 2 | Keep Moving

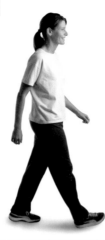

There is nothing better for energizing your entire body through movement than the simple act of walking. Last week you saw how easy it was to build 10 minutes a day into your routine. This week you'll just double that time to walk a total of 20 minutes per day.

CORE STABILITY   10 MINUTES

Repeat core stability from Week 1

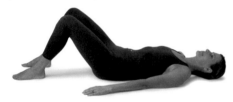

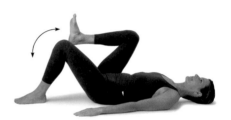

1. Lie on your back with knees bent, feet flat on the floor.

2. Press your lower back to the floor so there is not enough room to put your fingers between your spine and the floor. Hold your lower back in this position throughout the core stability exercises.

3. Lift your right knee up and down 5 times, keeping the foot 1 inch off the ground.

4. Repeat with the left knee. Do this exercise while slowly counting to 4. Slowly inhale while lifting the foot up. Slowly exhale while bringing the foot down to a count of 4, keeping the foot 1 inch off the ground.

New core stability for Week 2
1. Holding both knees up, feet off the ground, place the right foot on the floor and bring it back up. Repeat 5 times.

2. Repeat with the left foot. Hold the lower back against the floor the whole time. Do this exercise slowly while putting the foot down and exhaling. Slowly inhale while lifting the foot back up.

For more physical activities or relaxation techniques, please visit www.energizeyourlife.com.

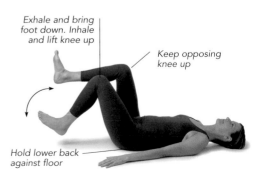

Exhale and bring foot down. Inhale and lift knee up

Keep opposing knee up

Hold lower back against floor

2 WEEK | Relax Deeper

STRETCHING   10 MIN

Stretching after physical activity will help prevent injuries and keep your body ready for more movement.

1. Standing on a belt, bend over and grab onto the belt as far down as you can reach.

2. Hold this position for 20 breaths. Build up to 50 breaths in 10-breath increments, gradually grasping lower on the belt.

3. Slowly come up from the stretch to begin the next exercise.

Keep your back straight. Bend from the hips, not from the back

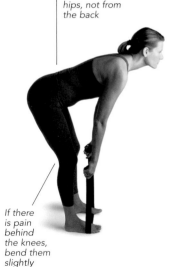

If there is pain behind the knees, bend them slightly

BREATH TRAINING: BASICS   10 MINUTES

The goal of this breathing exercise is to learn how to calm your breath. Slower breathing makes your brain chemistry shift from stress mode to relaxation mode. Research shows that, by slowing their breathing, people can control their heart rate, blood pressure and digestion.

1. Sit up straight in a chair and keep your head level. Gently exhale all of your air. Close the right nostril with the thumb of the right hand, and inhale slowly and deeply through the left nostril.

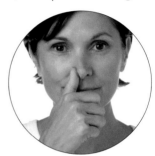

2. Close the left nostril with the ring finger (fourth finger), release the thumb and exhale through the right nostril.

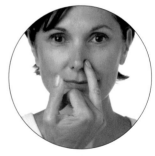

3. Inhale through the right nostril, then close it with the thumb and exhale through the left. Do 10 rounds.

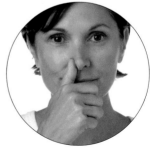

This technique is especially good for body-oriented people.

THE THREE-WEEK PLAN

Week 3: Plan for Life

What to expect

During Week 3 you will double your goal for walking. It may seem like a challenge to find the time, but as your energy level increases, you will find that you are actually able to get more done each day. You can bring lean red meat back into your diet and start using some powerful relaxation techniques.

As you enter the final phase of the Plan, you are already feeling like a new chapter of your life has begun. This week, you will put the finishing touches on a set of habits—new ways of eating, moving and relaxing—designed for maximum energy and health. You will use your increased energy to step up your movement program, you will eat more varied and protein-rich foods and you will learn a method of positive thinking that promotes all-around happiness.

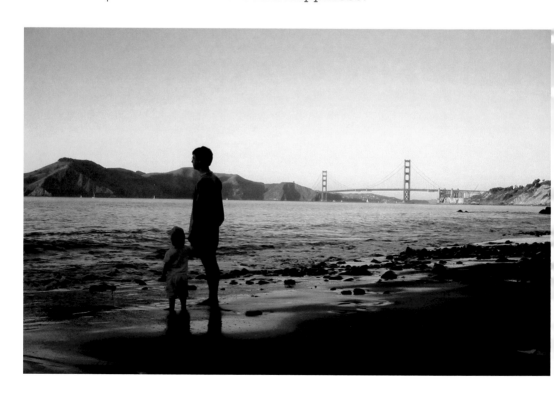

Wake-up

Drink 8-oz hot lemon water (recipe, page 44)

Begin core stability exercises (page 65)

Do positive thinking (page 67) or visualization training (page 49)

Low-fat dairy products are a good source of calcium and protein. You may be pleasantly surprised by what you find. For example, Italian parmesan cheese is made from low-fat milk.

Morning

Eat fruit and/or drink 8-oz protein shake or smoothie (recipe, page 44) OR eat 1-2 poached eggs with rye bread (recipe, page 54)

Eat 2-4 rice cakes

Consume 10-oz Matay Slimming Energy Drink

Take vitamin supplements (page 61)

Mid-morning

Warm up (jump up and down 5 times) and walk 20 minutes

Eat fruit and/or drink 8-oz protein shake/smoothie

Consume 10-oz Matay Slimming Energy Drink

Noon

Eat one 6-oz serving of poultry, fish or lean red meat or 1-2 eggs with salad and vegetable soup (recipe, page 44) OR eat 1 cup rice, quinoa or buckwheat and steamed vegetables (recipe, page 44)

Consume 10-oz Matay Slimming Energy Drink

Afternoon

Eat fruit and/or drink 8-oz protein shake or smoothie

Warm up (jump up and down 5 times) and walk 20 minutes After your walk, do the stretching postures (page 64)

Some people find that one 40-minute walk a day works better for their schedule.

Evening

Eat one 6-oz serving of poultry, fish or lean red meat with salad and vegetable soup OR eat 1 cup rice, quinoa or buckwheat and steamed vegetables

Before sleep

Drink 8-oz hot herbal tea

Do candle gazing (page 66) or breath training (page 67) or resting pose (page 48) and go to sleep

_{WEEK} 3 | Daily Food Choices

Items in red are new foods this week.

Beverages **Many** **servings**		Lemon water; purified water; herbal, green and maté teas Alcohol (optional): 1 glass of wine a day (up to 4 glasses a week)	Avoid: Soda and diet sodas, sweetened juices and drinks, alcohol; high-calorie coffee drinks
Fruit **Many** **servings**	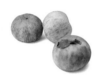	For better digestion, eat melons on their own, not with other fruit. Try a platter of fresh apple, mango, papaya, pineapple and grapefruit after a meal instead of dessert.	
Vegetables **Many** **servings**	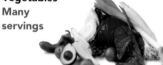	Eat a variety of vegetables in any combination. High in soluble fiber: peas, bok choy, yellow squash	
Grains **2 cups**		Rice: brown, basmati, jasmine, wild rice; rice cakes; rice-based breads Grains: quinoa, millet, amaranth, teff, kasha (roasted buckwheat), whole rye bread (2 slices)	Avoid: Refined grains as found in white bread, donuts, pasta
Legumes **2 cups**		Mung beans, bean sprouts, tofu, soybeans, lentils, miso, chick peas, adzuki beans, pinto beans, kidney beans, split peas, black-eyed peas, white beans, soy milk	Avoid: Any legume that causes intestinal discomfort. Soak beans in water for 8 hours to prevent gas. Drain, rinse and add fresh water to cook.
Fats and oils		Extra virgin olive oil: Up to 2 tablespoons Cold pressed flax oil: Up to 1 tablespoon	Avoid: Margarine, butter, hydrogenated fats and other oils

Flax oil is a healthy fat called omega-3 fat. It reduces the risk of heart attack and stroke, lowers blood pressure and relieves asthma and depression.

Condiments
As needed

Vegetable, seasoned or sea salt; apple cider, balsamic and rice vinegars; wheat-free tamari; all spices; miso; low-calorie mayonnaise; mustard

Avoid:
MSG, regular mayonnaise, artificial flavors, preservatives, sugary relishes, bottled salad dressings

---

Nuts and seeds
1-oz serving

Raw nuts: almond, pecan, hazelnut, Brazil, cashew, pine nuts, macadamia, pistachio, walnut
Raw seeds: sunflower, poppy, pumpkin, sesame and sesame butter

Avoid:
Peanuts and all nuts that are roasted, dry-roasted, canned or salted

---

Poultry and fish
6-oz serving
Eggs
2 eggs = 1 serving
Lean red meat
6-oz serving, once a week

Poultry: turkey, chicken, goose, guinea fowl, pheasant, duck
Fish: crab, shrimp, lobster, halibut, herring, mackerel, salmon, sardines
Meat: beef, veal, lamb, venison

Avoid:
Farmed fish, fish high in mercury (swordfish, tuna), meats high in saturated fat like bacon and ribs

---

Dairy
Low-fat hard cheese
2-oz serving
Low-fat yogurt
8-oz serving

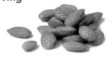

Cheeses: feta, gruyère, parmesan, mozzarella, romano, swiss
Dairy: low-fat cottage cheese or yogurt, kefir and buttermilk

Avoid:
All other dairy products
Substitute cow's milk with soy, rice or almond milk

Supplements

For more information on supplements, see page 70.

Whey protein powder (2 servings)
Multivitamin (one daily serving)
Vitamin C (500 mg)
Matay Slimming Energy Drink (three 10-oz servings)

More foods to avoid forever

No fatty red meat

No full-fat dairy
(replace with low-fat dairy or soy, rice or almond milk)

No chocolate, sugar, honey, molasses, jams, foods with preservatives or food coloring

No packaged, processed or fast foods

WEEK 3

WEEK 3 | Recipes

BREAKFAST & SNACKS

Potato Tofu Scramble

1 to 2 tbsp olive oil
2 garlic cloves, minced
½ onion, diced
8 oz firm tofu, cut into
    ½-inch pieces and drained
    for 15 minutes
2 eggs, whipped
2 large cooked potatoes,
    cut into ¾-inch pieces

Heat olive oil in a frying pan. Sauté the garlic and onion on high heat for 1 minute. Add the chopped tofu and continue cooking for 1 minute. Stir in the whipped eggs and then add the potatoes. Cover for 1 minute, then turn down the heat and uncover the pan. Stir and cook until the eggs are solid and any liquid has evaporated. Serve with Parmesan cheese, hot sauce, salsa or season with salt and pepper.

LUNCH & DINNER

Simple Greek Salad

1 English cucumber, cubed
1 cup tomatoes,
    cut into 1-inch cubes
¼ cup red onion, diced
1 each yellow and green peppers,
    cut into ½-inch pieces
½ to 1 cup whole, pitted black
    olives (optional)
½ cup soy feta cheese, crumbled
Dried Greek herb blend
Olive oil and lemon juice

Combine the vegetables and cheese. Sprinkle with herbs and drizzle with olive oil and lemon juice. Toss and serve.

Baked Salsa Chicken with Beans

1 15-oz can red kidney beans,
    rinsed and drained
1 cup mild salsa
2 garlic cloves, minced
1 lb skinless boneless chicken
    breasts, cut into 2-inch pieces

Preheat oven to 350 degrees. In a 13-inch x 9-inch baking pan, combine the beans, salsa and garlic. Add the chicken and baste with some of the salsa. Bake about 45 minutes, until the chicken is cooked. Stir the beans and baste the chicken midway through the baking. Serves 4.

Pesto Vegetables

2 cups broccoli,
    cut into 1-inch florets
1 red or green pepper,
    cut into 1-inch pieces
1 small eggplant,
    cut into 1-inch pieces
1 red onion,
    cut into 1-inch pieces
1 large carrot and/or parsnip,
    cut in ¼-inch diagonal slices
1 medium zucchini,
    cut into ½-inch slices
1 to 2 tbsp olive oil

Pesto

2 tbsp pine nuts or walnuts
1 cup fresh basil, packed
2 cloves of garlic
¼ cup extra virgin olive oil

Place the cut-up vegetables in a large bowl and add the olive oil. Stir to coat the vegetables, pour out onto a cookie sheet and broil for 10 minutes or until tender. Remove from the oven, pour the vegetables into a large bowl and toss with the pesto. Serve over buckwheat or soy pasta or brown rice.

Use whatever vegetables you have on hand. For variety try asparagus, cut into 2-inch pieces with the tough ends discarded; tomatoes, quartered; or yellow squash, cut into 1-inch pieces. Serves 4 to 6.

For more tasty recipes and nutritional information, please visit www.energizeyourlife.com.

Harvest Polka Dot Soup

1 to 2 tbsp extra virgin olive oil
2 cloves garlic, roughly chopped
1 medium white onion, quartered,
  with ends removed
1 tsp cinnamon
1 tsp nutmeg
1 tsp cumin
8 cups water
1 potato, cut into 1-inch pieces
1 sweet potato or yam,
  cut into 1-inch pieces
2 carrots, cut into 1-inch slices
1 parsnip, cut into 1-inch pieces
2 stalks celery, cut into 1-inch slices
2 tsp grated raw ginger
½ cup fresh orange juice (optional)
1 15-oz can black beans, rinsed
  and drained
Salt and pepper to taste

Heat the oil olive in a large pot.
Lightly sauté the garlic, onion and
the spices for 1 to 2 minutes.
Add 8 cups of water and all the
vegetables. Bring to a boil, turn
the heat down and simmer until
vegetables are tender, about
20 minutes. Cool and purée in a
blender. Pour the purée into the
pot to reheat and add the optional
orange juice. Add the black beans
and cook until heated. Salt and
pepper to taste. Serves 6.

EATING AWAY FROM HOME

Breakfast
Look for: Whole grain cereal,
rye-based breads, fresh fruits,
poached or boiled eggs

Avoid: Cereals high in fat or sugar
(most store bought breakfast
cereals), donuts, pastries, muffins,
croissants, butter, cream cheese,
fried eggs, ham, bacon, sausage,
hash browns

Salads
Look for: Fresh vegetables, beans,
fruit, boiled or poached eggs
Request dressing on the side and
use sparingly.

Avoid: Chicken or tuna salads
with mayonnaise, pre-dressed
pasta salads, coleslaw, marinated
vegetables, bacon bits, croutons,
macaroni, creamy salad dressings

Soups
Look for: Broth-based soup

Avoid: Cream-based soups
(clam chowder, cream of tomato)

Main dishes
Ask for a dish with less oil or
request to modify the dish to suit
your healthy eating habits. Opt
for poached, grilled, steamed or
roasted chicken, red meat or fish,
with steamed vegetables.

Dessert
Opt for fresh fruit or herbal tea.

Mexican
Look for: Grilled, baked or
sautéed meats, soft tortillas,
gazpacho soup, black bean soup,
salads, salsa, fajitas, burritos
without cheese

Avoid: Fried dishes, enchiladas,
cheese quesadillas, refried beans
(flavored with lard), fried tortilla
chips, nachos, tacos, sour cream,
chorizo, flan, sopapillas, fried
ice cream

Chinese
Look for: Baked, sautéed or
stir-fried, steamed or BBQ meats,
vegetables

Avoid: Fried (batter- or pan-fried),
crispy, sweet and sour, egg rolls
and spring rolls, lo mein, scallion
pancakes, Peking duck

Italian
Look for: Grilled, baked, sautéed
or roasted meats, medallions,
beans, seafood, primavera,
vegetables, fresh clam sauces,
olives, brown rice risottos

Avoid: Fried, pasta, cream sauces
(alfredo, carbonara), extra cheese,
parmigiana, pancetta, prosciutto,
pepperoni, salami, meatballs,
francese, Milanese, piccata

3 WEEK | Move into Energy

CONTINUE WALKING — 40 MINUTES

You may find that while movement used to seem like something you "ought to do," it now feels like something you need to do. Your body wants to move every day, so let it!

This week you will begin walking 40 minutes a day (in one session or two 20-minute sessions). If this causes excessive soreness, build towards your goal by starting at 20 minutes and increasing by 5 minutes a day until you reach 40. Your muscles will grow stronger to adapt to your new activity level.

STRETCHING — 10 MINUTES

Repeat stretching from Week 2
1. Standing on a belt, bend over and grab onto the belt as far down as you can reach.

2. Hold this position for 20 breaths. Build up to 50 breaths in 10-breath increments, gradually grasping lower on the belt.

3. Slowly come up from the stretch to begin the next exercise.

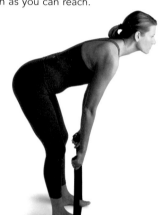

New stretching for Week 3
Repeat this same exercise sitting on the floor, bending forward to grab the belt around the front of the feet. Work up to 50 breaths. Try to do most of your stretching on the exhaled breath.

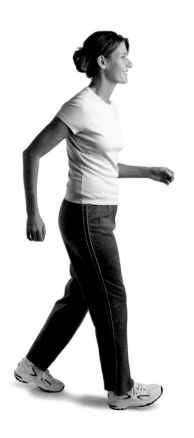

Keep your back straight. Bend from the hips, not from the back

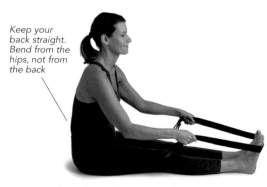

For more physical activities, please visit www.energizeyourlife.com.

Repeat core stability from Week 1

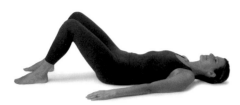

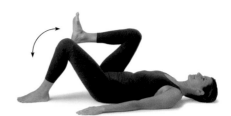

1. Lie on your back with knees bent, feet flat on the floor.

2. Press your lower back to the floor so there is not enough room to put your fingers between your spine and the floor. Hold your lower back in this position throughout the core stability exercises.

3. Lift your right knee up and down 5 times, keeping the foot 1 inch off the ground.

4. Repeat with the left knee. Do this exercise while slowly counting to 4. Slowly inhale while lifting the foot up. Slowly exhale while bringing the foot down to a count of 4, keeping the foot 1 inch off the ground.

Repeat core stability from Week 2

1. Holding both knees up, feet off the ground, place the right foot on the floor and bring it back up. Repeat 5 times.

2. Repeat with the left foot. Hold the lower back against the floor the whole time. Do this exercise slowly while putting the foot down and exhaling. Slowly inhale while lifting the foot back up.

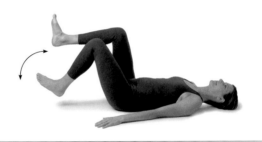

New core stability for Week 3

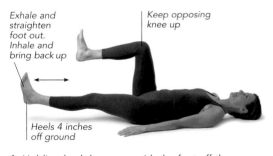

Exhale and straighten foot out. Inhale and bring back up

Keep opposing knee up

Heels 4 inches off ground

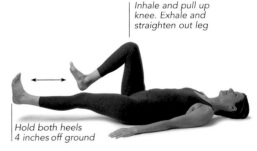

Inhale and pull up knee. Exhale and straighten out leg

Hold both heels 4 inches off ground

1. Holding both knees up with the feet off the ground, straighten the right leg with the right heel 4 inches off the ground and bring it back up to the bent knee position. Repeat 5 times.

2. Repeat with the left leg. Do this exercise slowly while straightening the foot out and exhaling. Slowly inhale while lifting the foot up.

1. With both legs straight and the heels 4 inches from the floor, pull the right knee up to the chest and then push it straight back out. Repeat 5 times.

2. Repeat with the left leg. Do this exercise slowly while bringing the knee up and inhaling. Slowly exhale while straightening the leg out.

WEEK 3 | Relax into the Future

Even people with a lot of experience with relaxation techniques will tell you: It's not always easy. Your mind is constantly in motion, shifting gears from moment to moment. The important thing is to be patient. Even if you have days when you can't relax, stick with it. You are getting the benefits of these techniques just by taking the time each day to try.

You have learned to give your body what it needs and to stay away from harmful and energy-draining foods. Round out your energized lifestyle by treating your mind to healthy thoughts. This week, you will nourish your inner self with affirmations: positive words and images. With them, you can encourage yourself to stick with the Plan at the same time as you improve your mood and attitude.

CANDLE GAZING   5 MINUTES

Candle gazing teaches you to relax and focus.

1. Sit on the floor or on a chair with a candle lit in front of you at eye level.

2. Breathe in a relaxed way, keeping your eyes on the flame. Do not blink your eyes; keep them open and tears may naturally begin to flow. As you stare at the flame, thoughts will come to mind. When this happens, let go of the thought and bring your attention back to the flame. Repeat this each time your mind wanders: just come back to the candle.

3. After five minutes, blow out the candle and close your eyes. This is a very relaxing method to practice just before bed.

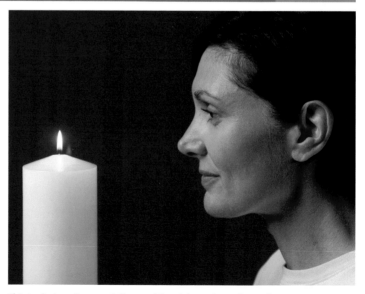

This technique is especially good for vision-oriented people.

As you go through life, every thought, perception and feeling is expressed in your body as a chemical reaction. Negative thoughts produce stress hormones that reduce your energy and ability to heal. By intentionally bringing positive thoughts into your mind, you can change the whole system to work in your favor. Creating positive thoughts changes your body chemistry and improves your well-being.

1. Think of something about yourself you would like to improve. Write it at the top of a piece of paper (for example, firmer tummy).

2. Think of a way you can achieve this goal. Write this down as a positive "I" statement about what you will do to get there (for example, "I will stick to the Plan and eat five servings of fresh vegetables every day" instead of "I will not eat ice cream").

3. Put the paper in a prominent yet private place where you will see it every day. Read the goal and how you will achieve it aloud five times every day (for example, stick the note on your bathroom mirror).

This technique is especially good for auditory-oriented people.

This week the breath training focuses on regulating the breath with timed inhalation and exhalation. As you learn to make the breath slower, you will gain control over your nervous system and learn to control the "stress" signals that raise blood pressure, speed up the heart and constrict circulation.

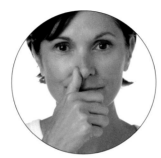

1. Sit up straight in a chair and keep your head level. Gently exhale all of your air. Close the right nostril with the thumb of the right hand, and inhale slowly and deeply through the left nostril. Start by taking 3 seconds to inhale, and work up to a count of 10 seconds.

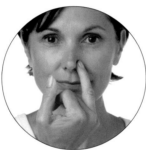

2. Close the left nostril with the ring finger (fourth finger), release the thumb and exhale through the right nostril. Start by taking 3 seconds to exhale, and work up to a count of 10 seconds.

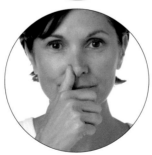

3. Inhale through the right nostril, then close it with the thumb and exhale through the left, timing to a count of 3 seconds and working up to a count of 10 seconds. This cycle of two breaths makes one round. Do 10 rounds.

This technique is especially good for body-oriented people.

WEEK 3

For more relaxation techniques, please visit www.enerergizeyourlife.com

Beyond Week 3: Now What?

Congratulations on completing your Three-Week Plan. Energy, weight loss and a good attitude are your rewards—they belong to you. They replace fatigue, being overweight and feeling stressed out. In order to hold onto the Plan's benefits, you have to do just one thing: stick with it. Remember that you have the force of habit on your side: once you establish the Plan as your daily pattern, it will become easier to follow. If you lose focus, just return to this book and remind yourself of the unhealthy habits you left behind and the energizing choices you now make—every day!

WHAT YOU EAT

Eating well and enjoying your food actually extends life and improves your health. Keep this book in your kitchen and flip through it before going shopping. The food we recommend here, known as the "Mediterranean-style diet," is rich in plant foods and fish, low in meat and dairy products and has a high ratio of monounsaturated to polyunsaturated fats. It decreases body weight and blood pressure and regulates blood sugar and hormone levels.

WHAT YOU DO

After three weeks of walking, stretching and core stability training, your body is beginning to change. Continue this program for another three weeks. The goal is to become physically dependent on exercise. Soon, a day without activity will feel wrong to you; you will need to move. And you will want to add to your program, either by extending your time, by adding weight training or taking up a ball sport, bowling or even ballroom dancing. The main goal is to find a comfortable yet challenging level and have fun as you get fit.

WHAT YOU FEEL

Now that you have made room in your day for relaxation, you will start to feel calmer overall. Remember to seek out relaxing activities like massage, music and reading. You will discover that de-stressing is easier once you find techniques that fit your individual nature. When relaxation becomes a habit like brushing your teeth, it won't be a chore; it will feel like a necessity for your inner well-being. You'll see the rewards in your health, and the people around you will benefit from your increased calmness.

Healthy Food Substitutes

Potato chips
Baked bean chips, rice crackers, raw nuts

Candy bars
Raw nuts and dried fruit

Soda
Juice spritzer

Dessert
Fruit and low-fat cheese platter

Wheat-based pasta
Rice, buckwheat or soy noodles

Cream
Low-fat yogurt

Butter, lard, margarine, shortening
Olive oil

Milk
Low-fat yogurt, soy, almond or rice milk

Sugar, pancake syrup, sweetener
Pure maple syrup

Bread
Rice crackers, rye or rice-based breads

Fitness Expert

Fitness Expert is a combination of two devices: a "Body Analyzer" and "Calorie Tracker." These medical-grade devices will accurately measure and record your daily caloric burn as you sleep, work, relax and exercise. The Body Analyzer is an electronic device that will tell you your hydration (water) level, your lean muscle mass and your body fat. The Calorie Tracker is a sophisticated calorie-monitoring device and is not to be confused with simple pedometers. More information is available at www.FitnessExpert.com.

The 1-in-10 rule
Treat yourself by going "off the plan" 1 out of 10 meals. Go out for dinner and eat what you want or share a dessert with a friend.

Don't shop when you are hungry
Shopping when you are hungry is a bad idea. You will impulse-buy unhealthy foods, including snack foods. Shop after a meal instead.

Avoid sugars and breads
Everyone loves a sweet taste. Instead of sugar and bread, eat yogurt, nuts, fruit and cheese.

Eat well
Always eat breakfast. Chew your food thoroughly: the more you taste it, the more satisfying your food will be. Don't chew and read. When you eat, sit down at a table and just eat!

Walk with others
Energize your walking by joining a walking club in your community. Sign up for a walkathon to meet people or fundraise.

Join the party
Don't feel left out— have your healthy drink in a fancy glass and join in the toasting!

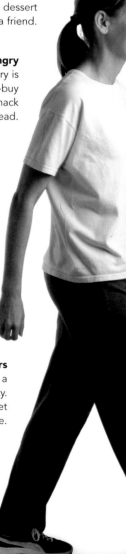

Helpful Products

Here are some healthful products that will help you on your way as you begin your journey to an energized life. To order the following products, go to www.quixtar.com

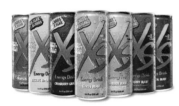

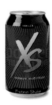

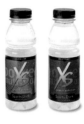

XS™ Energy Drinks

A low-carb, sugar-free blast of energy that delivers a powerful punch of B vitamins to help boost mental and physical energy.

XS™ Power Nutrition Shakes

Ready-to-drink with 35 grams of protein and 4-5 grams of carbs to help make protein-loading easy, delicious and nutritious. Contains exclusive C-Lenium Blend to help protect against harmful free radicals.

XS™ Power Nutrition Sports Drinks

Replenish, regain, renew with these outstanding sports drinks. They contain electrolytes, selenium and an exclusive B-Lenium Blend for energy production.

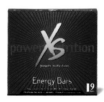

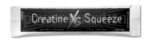

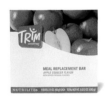

XS™ Power Nutrition Energy Bars

Help fuel muscle recovery and boost energy with 15 grams of protein and just 7 net available carbs in each scrumptious bar with excellent antioxidant protection.

XS™ Power Nutrition Creatine Squeeze

Before exercise, its patented stabilized delivery system delivers 2.5 grams of protein, enabling you to exercise at a higher intensity and, possibly, for a longer period of time.

TRIM ADVANTAGE® Meal Replacement Bars

These luscious bars provide nutrients when you're on the go, giving you 15-16 grams of protein, fiber and one third of the daily value of 24 vitamins and minerals.

or www.xsgear.com. Be sure to also visit www.energizeyourlife.com for more tips and helpful products.

7-Day Detox Miracle, 2nd edition
By Peter Bennett, N.D., and Stephen Barrie, N.D. Prima Lifestyles, 2001. Revitalize your mind and body with this safe and effective life-enhancing program.

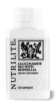

NUTRILITE® Glucosamine
A key building block for semi-fluids that lubricate joints. There's clinical evidence that people have significant improvement in joint function and build joint cartilage supplementing with 1,500 mg of glucosamine HCL per day.

NUTRILITE® Muscle Rescue
Keep moving with the natural way to get temporary relief from minor aches and pains—and occasional muscle stiffness associated with strenuous exercise.

NUTRILITE® Valerian and Hops
A natural herbal blend to help you sleep! The valerenic acid in valerian has been clinically proven to help people fall asleep faster and stay asleep longer.

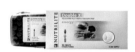

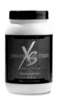

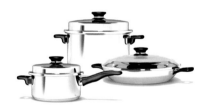

NUTRILITE® Double X Vitamin/Mineral/Phytonutrient
Packed with higher levels of the vitamins and minerals that most of us don't get from our diets. It's supercharged with concentrates from 16 natural plant sources and it contains very high levels of phytonutrients. The result is energy you can feel all day.

XS™ Power Nutrition Whey Protein Powder
Delivers 50 grams of natural whey protein and less than 5 grams of net available carbs. Excellent for toning muscle and building muscle mass.

iCook Products
Premium-grade materials and precision manufacturing provide years of superb cooking performance and durability. Stack cooking capability saves space, time and fuel costs. Improved heat distribution and ergonomic design makes iCook products easy to use.

Credits

Content development, information
architecture and design: Hot Studio, Inc.
Creative director: Maria Giudice
Art director and designer: Piper Murakami
Information architect, designer: Renee Anderson
Producer: Hazel Sharpe

Hot Studio, Inc.
848 Folsom Street, Suite 201
San Francisco, CA 94107
415.284.7250
info@hotstudio.com

Editorial: Peter Bennett, Stephen Barrie, Steve Muller
Proofreaders: Ann-Marie Metten, Sarah Vanderveen
Photography: Lisa Keenan Photography, Emeryville, CA
Photo assistants: Kelly Powers, Shana Lopes
Photo production: Dave Shultz, Don Haaga
Prop stylist: Carol Hacker
Food stylist: Pouke
Food stylist assistant: Jeffrey Larsen
Recipes: Louise Clausson, Paul Patterson of Conceptual
Development Group (www.c-d-g.com), Piper Murakami
Product photography courtesy of Quixtar Inc.
©2005 Quixtar Inc. All rights reserved.

Special thank you: Linda Stone, Dr. Stephanie
Trenciansky, David Vanderveen, Greg Duncan,
Scott Coon, Wynn Gmitroski
Additional thank you: Henrik Olsen, Cheryn Flanagan,
Anita Liu, Kevin Allen, Jeannette Muzio, Arlene
Utsurogi, Marcus Pape, Diane VanHoven, Arwen O'Reilly
Inspiring loved ones: Avalon, Nur, Kirsten, Meera,
Mason, Angelica

Printing: Hemlock Printers, Canada